Ultrasound Teaching Manual

The Basics of Performing and
Interpreting Ultrasound Scans

Matthias Hofer

2nd Edition

406 images with 741 illustrations

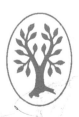

2005

Georg Thieme Verlag

Stuttgart • New York

Library of Congress Cataloging-in-Publication Data is available from the publisher.

Matthias Hofer, M.D., MPH

Head, Medical Education Pilot Project
Institutes of Diagnostic Radiology & Anatomy II
H. Heine-University
P.O. Box 10 10 07
40001 Duesseldorf, Germany

Images Obstetrics & Gynecology by:

Tatjana Reihs, M.D.

Dept. of Obstetrics & Gynecology
H. Heine-University
P.O. Box 10 10 07
40001 Duesseldorf, Germany

1st	German edition	1995
1st	Japanese edition	1995
1st	Dutch edition	1996
2nd	German edition	1997
1st	Greek edition	1997
3rd	German edition	1999
2nd	Japanese edition	2000
1st	Italian edition	2001
1st	French edition	2001
4th	German edition	2002
1st	Russian edition	2003
1st	Portugese edition	2004
1st	Spanish edition	2004

© 2005 Georg Thieme Verlag,
Rüdigerstraße 14, D-70469 Stuttgart, Germany
Thieme New York, 333 Seventh Avenue,
New York, N.Y. 10001 U.S.A.
Website: http://www.thieme.com

Typesetting by Inger Jürgens, Düsseldorf

Printed in Germany by Hohnrath Creativ Druck,
Korschenbroich

ISBN 1-58890-279-X (TNY)
ISBN 3-13-111042-2 (GTV)

Important Note: Medicine is an ever-changing science undergoing continual development. Research and clinical experience are continually expanding our knowledge; in particular our knowledge of proper treatment and drug therapy. Insofar as this book mentions any dosage or application, readers may rest assured that the authors, editors, and publishers have made every effort to ensure that such references are in accordance with *the state of knowledge at the time of production of the book.*

Nevertheless, this does not involve, imply, or express any guarantee or responsibility on the part of the publishers in respect of any dosage instructions and forms of application stated in the book. *Every user is requested to examine carefully* the manufacturer's leaflets accompanying each drug and to check, if necessary in consultation with a physician or specialist, whether the dosage schedules mentioned therein or the contraindications stated by the manufacturers differ from the statements made in the present book. Such examination is particularly important with drugs that are either rarely used or have been newly released on the market. Every dosage schedule or every form of application used is entirely at the user's own risk and responsibility. The authors and publishers request every user to report to the publishers any discrepancies or inaccuracies noticed.

If errors in this work are found after publication, errata will be posted at www.thieme.com on the product description page.

Some of the product names, patents, and registered designs referred to in this book are in fact registered trademarks or proprietary names, even though specific reference to this fact is not always made in the text. Therefore, the appearence of a name without designation as proprietary is not to be construed as a representation by the publisher that it is in the public domain.

How can you use this workbook optimally?
By working through the chapters separately, you can benefit from several methodical and didactic features:

Rapid search ...
- For a chapter – you will find a tab for each chapter on page 5,
- For tough quiz questions and going more in-depth – also explained on page 5,
- For cross-referenced figures – the numeration corresponds to the page the figures appear on, for example **Fig. 36.2** is on page 36,
- For an explanatory figure or diagram of the text – they are marked in light blue at the appropriate site of the accompanying text and are almost always on the same page, thus avoiding unnecessary browsing,
- For an annotated number – marked bold in the accompanying text or found on the unfolded back cover flap (the same number for all pages of the entire book),

- For terms in the index – on page 116 (or even on pages 4 and 5),
- For normal values and checklists – provided on laminated, water-resistant, pocket-sized cards.

Why is this book called a "workbook"?
Every page can be used as a quiz to test your knowledge. Since the diagrams are annotated by numbers and not by names, you can check every diagram to find the sonographically shown structures you are familiar with and those you do not yet know. The quiz questions and drawing exercises have a similar purpose.

In this way, you can familiarize yourself with several efficient study methods that allow your newly acquired knowledge to become your long-term knowledge fast – even though this process demands your active participation. I wish you success and lots of fun!

Matthias Hofer, November 2004

List of Abbreviations

A.	Artery	ERCP	Endoscopic retrograde cholangiopancreaticography	mW	Milliwatt
Aa.	Arteries			NB	Newborn
AC	Abdominal circumference (fetus)	ESWL	Extracorporeal shock wave lithotripsy	NHL	Non-Hodgkin lymphoma
AG	Adrenal gland	FL	Femur length (fetus)	NPO	non per os (fasting)
AIUM	American Institute of Ultrasound in Medicine	FNH	Focal nodular hyperplasia	NT	Nuchal Translucency (fetus)
		FOD	Fronto-occipital diameter (fetus)	PPI	Parenchyma-pelvic index
AO	Aorta			PT	Preterm newborn
ASD	Atrial septal defect	GIT	Gastrointestinal tract	PW	Pulsed wave (Doppler)
BC	Bronchial carcinoma	HC	Head circumference	RCS	Renal collecting system
BE	Barium enema	HCG	Human chorionic gonadotropin	RI	Resistive index
BPD	Biparietal diameter (fetus)			RT	Renal transplant
b/w	Black-white (B-mode) sonography	HJ	Hip joint	SAS	Subarachnoid CSF space
		IHW	Width of the SAS in the interhemispheric fissure	SCW	Sinocortical width of the SAS
CCD	Chorionic cavity diameter			SD	Standard deviation
CCE	Cholecystectomy	IUD	Intrauterine device	SLE	Systemic lupus erythematosus
CCW	Craniocerebral width of the external subarachnoid CSF space	IVC	Inferior vena cava		
		IVF	In vitro fertilization	SMA	Superior mesenteric artery
		IVP	Intravenous pyelogram	TGA	Transposition of the great arteries
CHI	Contrast harmonic imaging	LA	Lower abdomen		
CRL	Crown-rump length (fetus)	Lig.	Ligament	THI	Tissue harmonic imaging
CSF	Cerebrospinal fluid	LN	Lymph node	UA	Upper abdomen
CT	Computed tomography	M.	Muscle	UB	Urinary bladder
CW	Continuous wave (Doppler)	MA	Mid-abdomen	V.	Vein
d_{AO}	Diameter of the aorta	MCL	Medioclavicular line	Vv.	Veins
DGC	Depth gain compensation	MHz	Megahertz (frequency unit)	VCUG	Voiding cystourethrogram
d_{VC}	Diameter of the vena cava	Mm.	Muscles	Vol_{UB}	Volume of the urinary bladder
EP	Ectopic pregnancy	MRI	Magnetic resonance imaging	VSD	Ventricular septal defect
				YS	Yolk sac

Contents

Where Do I Find a Particular Chapter?

Do you want more than "just reading"?
Experience has shown that readers and course participants get the greatest benefit from this book by trying to draw the standard sections with sportsmanlike ambition from memory and to solve the quiz questions alone. You will be surprised how fast the new knowledge becomes your long-term knowledge. To find the relevant pages easily, the quiz headings are marked in **blue** in the list of contents and the pages bear a blue tab laterally:

Are you interested in pediatrics?
We also placed tabs for easy finding of pages with pediatric content. They are just above the lower corner of the outer margin of the corresponding pages and appear as shown here:
They are found on pages 47, 48, 51–53, 56, 59, 63, 66, 67, 72, 91–98, 101, 104, 105

Image Formation

Sonographic images are generated by sound waves – not by X-rays – which are sent by a transducer into the human body and are reflected in it. In abdominal sonography, the frequencies used generally are between 2.5 and 5.0 MHz (see page 9).

The primary condition enabling sound wave reflection are so-called "impedance jumps," which occur at the interface between two tissues with different sound transmissions (interfaces in **Fig. 6.2**). It is interesting to note that different soft tissues show rather minor differences in the transmission of sound (**Tab. 6.1**). Only air and bone are marked by massively different sound transmission in comparison with soft tissues.

For this reason, sonographic units can be operated with a preselected medium frequency of 1540 m/sec for a calculation of the origin ("depth") of the echo without any major misconstruction. The processor computes the depth of origin of the echo from the registered temporal difference between emission of the sound impulse and return of the echo. Echoes from tissues close to the transducer (**A**) arrive earlier (t_A) than echoes from deeper tissues (t_B, t_C in **Fig. 6.2a**). The medium frequency is strictly theoretical since the receiver does not know which type of tissue was traversed.

Sound Transmission in Human Tissue		
Air	331 m/s	
Liver	1549 m/s	
Spleen	1566 m/s	$\overline{m} = 1540$ m/s
Muscle	1568 m/s	
Bone	3360 m/s	

Tab. 6.1

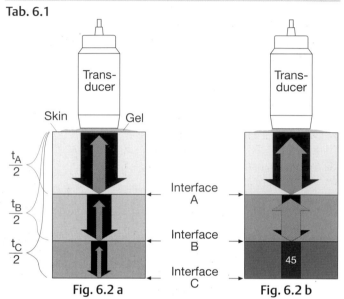

Fig. 6.2 a   Fig. 6.2 b

Which Component of the Sound Waves Is Reflected?

Fig. 6.2a shows three tissue blocks traversed by sound waves that barely differ in their sound velocity (indicated by similar grey values). Each interface only reflects a small portion of the original sound waves (↓) as echo (↑). The diagram on the right shows a larger impedance jump at the interface A between the different tissues (**Fig. 6.2b**). This increases the proportion of reflected sound waves (↑) in comparison to the tissues illustrated at left. However, what happens if the sound waves hit air in the stomach or a rib? This causes so-called "total reflection," as illustrated at interface B (**Fig. 6.2b**). The transducer does not detect any residual

sound waves to generate an image. Instead, the total reflection creates an acoustic shadow (**45**).

Conclusion: Intestinal or pulmonary air and bone are impenetrable by sound waves, precluding any imaging distal to these structures. Therefore the challenge is to work around these structures with the transducer. To this end, the pressure applied on the transducer (see page 17) and also the air-displacing gel between the surface of the transducer and the skin (see page 18) play a significant role.

From a "Snowstorm" to an Image ...

Don't get discouraged if at first you only make out a blinding "snowstorm" on the sonographic image. You will be surprised how soon you will recognize the sonographic morphology of individual organs and vessels. **Figure 6.3** shows two round polyps (**65**) in the gallbladder (**14**).

The surrounding grey "snowstorm" corresponds to the hepatic parenchyma (**9**), which is traversed by hepatic vessels (**10**, **11**). How can you quickly work out which structures in the image appear bright and which are dark? The key lies in the concept of echogenicity (see page 7).

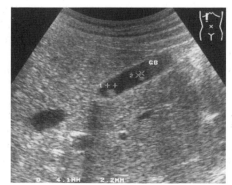

Fig. 6.3 a

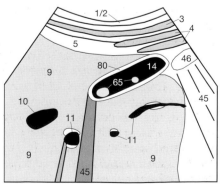

Fig. 6.3 b

What Does the Term "Echogenicity" Mean?

Tissues or organs with many intrinsic impedance jumps produce many echoes and appear **"echogenic" = bright**. In contrast, tissue and organs with few impedance jumps appear **"hypoechoic" = dark**.

Consequently, homogeneous fluids (blood, urine, bile, CSF, pericardial and pleural fluid) without impedance jumps appear **"anechoic" = black**.

The number of impedance jumps does not depend on the physical density (= mass/volume); a fatty liver can be used as good illustration.

In this unenhanced CT (**Fig. 7.1a**), the parenchyma of a fatty liver (9) appears darker (i.e., less dense) than hepatic vessels or normal liver (**Fig. 7.1b**). This is a result of the decreased density of fat in comparison to normal liver tissue.

Sonographically, the fatty deposits increase the impedance jumps (**Fig. 7.1c**) in comparison to normal liver tissue (**Fig. 7.1d**). Consequently, sonography shows the fatty liver more echogenic (brighter) despite its markedly decreased physical density.

A Common Misunderstanding

What do physicians mean when they refer to a dense liver? It reflects either sloppy language or ignorance. In contrast to radiographic methods, which visualize physical densities, sonography visualizes differences in sound velocities (impedance jumps), which are unrelated to physical density.

Please use the following terms:	These appear anechoic (= black):
Hyperechoic (= bright) **Hypoechoic (= dark)** **Anechoic (= black)**	Blood, urine, bile, CSF, pericardial or pleural effusion, ascites, cysts

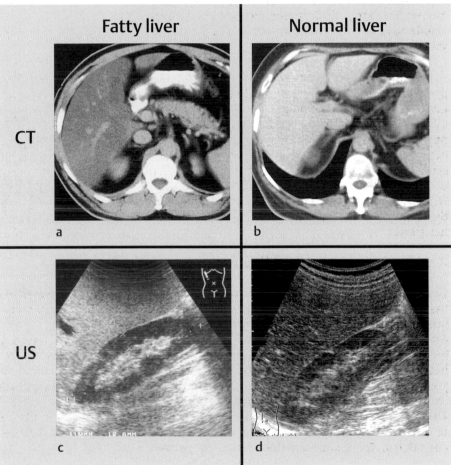

Fig. 7.1

Production and Frequencies of Sound Waves

The sonographic image begins with mechanical oscillations of crystals that have been excited by electric pulses, called the "piezoelectric effect." These oscillations are emitted as sound waves from the crystals. The reverse takes place when sound waves are received. Several crystals are assembled to form a transducer, from which pulsed sound waves of different frequencies stated in MHz are emitted. A "3.75 MHz" transducer does not exclusively emit pressure waves (= sound waves) with the frequency of 3.75 MHz; that is just the stated median frequency (= **"center frequency"**). In reality, such a transducer may emit sound wave frequencies between 2 and 6 MHz.

So-called **"multifrequency transducers"** have the additional capability to increase or decrease this center frequency and the surrounding bandwidth. In thin patients or children, for instance, the bandwidth can be increased to 4–8 MHz with a center frequency of 6 MHz to achieve better spatial resolution. However, this is achieved at the cost of less depth penetration of the sound waves.

In very obese patients, the use of lower frequencies (e.g., 1–5 MHz with a center frequency of 2.5 MHz) can be appropriate to achieve the necessary penetration, but by sacrificing resolution (see page 9). Newer methods use frequency shifts or harmonic frequencies of the fundamental frequency for image formation (see page 11).

Operating Sonographic Equipment

The operative elements on sonographic units are quite similar in function and arrangement, even among units from different vendors. It therefore should suffice to present the panel of one particular unit, which should also serve to introduce the relevant technical terms.

Most units have the stop–start button (E) in the lower right corner of the panel (Fig. 8.1) to freeze dynamic images. It is recommended to rest one finger of the left hand always on this button to minimize any delay in freezing the desired image. Before you begin, do not forget to enter the patient's name (A, B) for proper identification. The buttons for changing program (C) or transducer (D) are usually found on the upper half of the control panel. Programs with optimized parameters for frequency range, transducer, depth penetration, etc. can be stored in advance, allowing simple and fast switching between the organs to be examined, e.g., from the thyroid gland to the abdomen.

The overall amplification (gain) of the received echoes is controlled by the gain knob (F), which usually is larger than the other knobs. The amplification of echoes received from different depths can be selectively adjusted with slide-pots (G) to compensate for depth-related signal loss. In many units, magnification or visualized depth (= range) can be adjusted to the desired needs in small increments (H).

It requires some practice to operate the trackball (I) with the left hand to place the dot or range markers (calipers) in the desired position. In general, this must be preceded by activating one of the measurement modes (J) or the annotation mode (K). To make review of the images easier for others, the appropriate body marker (L) can be selected to mark the position of the transducer on the image before printing (M). The remaining functions vary among the machines of different vendors and are learned best by operating the unit in clinical practice.

Fig. 8.1: Console / Keyboard

A	Begin a new patient
B	Enter name (ID)
C	Menu selection
D	Change of transducer
E	Freeze
F	Gain
G	Depth gain compensation (DGC)
H	Image depth / field of view
I	Track ball for positioning the dot or range markers
J	Measurements
K	Annotations ("comments")
L	Body marker ("where was the transducer placed?")
M	Image recording / printer

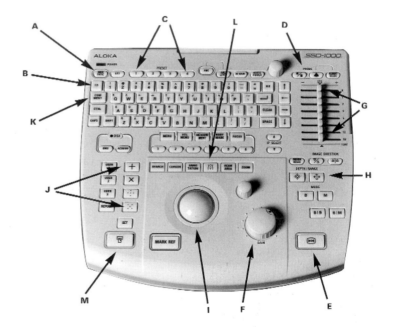

Specification of a Sonographic Unit

Besides price and image quality, user-friendliness should be considered when purchasing a sonographic unit. With only one exclusive inlet plug for a transducer, as often found on small units, it can be quite cumbersome when frequently different types of transducers are used (see page 9).

In view of the increasing digitalization in hospitals and physician offices, it is advisable to test the new unit for several days for compatibility with the existing data storage system. Thus, the invariably arising unexpected problems can be preemptively addressed by the vendor's customer service and subsequent disappointment or time-consuming upgrading avoided. To create a patient-friendly environment, it is advisable to install an additional monitor in the field of view of the lying patient, for instance in a corner of the examination room, to provide an opportunity for explaining the findings during the study. This small investment can improve the physician-patient relationship and the reputation of the hospital or office.

Not only pediatric examinations (though they gain the most) benefit from a unit with digital storage (cine loop) of adequate capacity that enables flashbacks for two (or more) seconds after freezing. With this option, images can be recorded on restless patients (or after slow freezing of the dynamic image) and optimal images selected or measurements taken without repeating the image acquisition. This option is now also available for smaller real-time units.

Selection of Sonographic Equipment

Besides large color Doppler units, additional sonographic units equipped with connections for several multifrequency transducers have been proven useful. They should be mobile so they can be moved easily from the sonography suite to other locations in the hospital (e.g., intensive care unit) (Fig. 9.1).

Precautions should be taken when transporting the sonographic unit. The transducers should be firmly attached to their haltering so that dangling transducer cables cannot be caught on doorknobs, stretchers, etc. Avoid dropping the transducers on the floor, since replacing a damaged transducer can be quite expensive. For the same reason, the transducer should never be left unattended on the patient's abdomen when the examination is interrupted, for instance by a phone call. Placing the transducers in the haltering with the cable hanging avoids unnecessary pinching or kinking where the cable enters the transducer (with a risk of broken wires in the cable).

Types of Transducers

Of the many types of transducers, only the applications of the three most important ones will be described here (endovaginal transducers, see page 75).

The **linear array transducer** emits parallel sound waves and produces a rectangular image. The width of the image and the number of scan lines are constant at all tissue levels (Fig. 9.2a). Linear array transducers have the advantage of a good near-field resolution, and are primarily used with high frequencies (5.0–10.0 MHz) for evaluating soft tissues and the thyroid gland. Their disadvantage is the large contact surface, leading to artifacts due to air gaps between skin and transducer when applied to a curved body contour.

Furthermore, acoustic shadowing (45) as caused by ribs, lungs or intestinal air can deteriorate the image. Consequently, linear array transducers are rarely used for visualizing thoracic or abdominal organs.

A **sector transducer** produces a fan-like image that is narrow near the transducer and increases in width with deeper penetration (Fig. 9.2b). This type of transducer has become established primarily in cardiology with frequencies of 2.0–3.0 MHz, which enable deeper penetration. Due to the fan-like propagation of the sound waves, the heart can be well visualized from a small intercostal window without interfering sound shadowing from the ribs. The disadvantages of these transducers are the poor resolution in the near field and decreasing line density in the far field, with corresponding decreasing resolution. Moreover, finding the desired image plane is more difficult and takes some practice.

The **curved or convex array transducer** is a combination of both preceding types (Fig. 9.2c). The shape of the monitor image resembles a coffee filter and combines a good near-field resolution with a relatively good far-field resolution. The major advantage of the slightly curved contact surface is the ability to displace interfering intestinal air outside the image plane (see page 17). For this type of transducer, however, decreasing resolution with increasing depth and, depending on the contact location, acoustic shadowing behind the ribs have to be tolerated. This type is predominantly used in abdominal sonography with frequencies from 2.5 MHz (very obese patients) to 5.0 MHz (slim patients). The average (center) frequency is at 3.5 to 3.75 MHz. Remember that higher sound frequencies have better resolution but less penetration.

Mnemonic: If loud music is coming from your neighbor's apartment, which tones do you hear? The basses, since they can penetrate the walls, proving the wider range (better penetration) of low frequencies. See page 7.

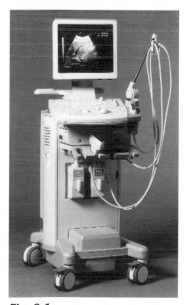

Fig. 9.1

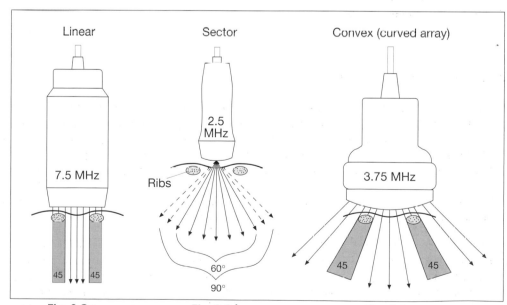

Fig. 9.2 a   Fig. 9.2 b   Fig. 9.2 c

Panoramic Imaging (SieScape®)

New high-performance image processors can merge the display of sonographic images captured by moving the transducer slowly and continuously over an entire body region of interest. With some practice, impressive and undistorted images with a measuring accuracy for distance of 1 - 3% can even be generated from a curved body surface.

Figure 10.1 shows a sagittal sonographic section with massive pleural effusion **(69)**, compression atelectasis of the lung **(47)** and subhepatic **(9)** anechoic ascites **(68)** inundating intestinal loops **(46)**.

Figure 10.2 illustrates the position of the placenta **(94)** relative to the fetus. The high contrast resolution even allows the evaluation of the interface between fetal liver **(9)** and lung **(47)**.

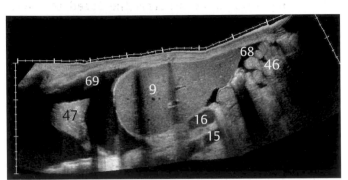

Fig. 10.1

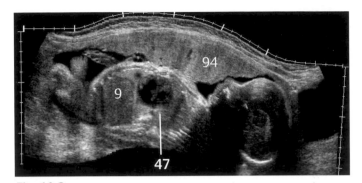

Fig. 10.2

(with kind permission of Drs. CF Dietrich and D Becker, from "Farbduplexsonography des Abdomens" Schnetztor-Verlag, Konstanz)

3-D Display

Especially in obstetrics, the three-dimensional display of the fetal facial features improves the diagnosis of malformations, for instance a cleft lip or palate. This technique can now display the fetal physiognomy with amazing accuracy **(Fig. 10.3)**.

Of course, conventional sonographic sections can also detect skeletal and other malformations (see page 89), but their display is less impressive and convincing than in the three-dimensional display.

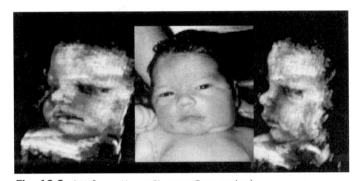

Fig. 10.3 (Wofgang Krzos, Siemens Corporation)

Photopic® Imaging

Since sonographic examinations are usually performed in darkened rooms, the examiner relies on scotopic perception with the retinal rods, which have sensitivities from 0.0001 to 10 cd/m². This "black-white" perception restricts the differentiation to 20 to 60 grey values, depending on the intensity of the ambient illumination and on the dark adaptation and vigilance of the examiner. The spatial resolution of the retina is relatively poor under these conditions.

In contrast, the photopic color perception of the retinal cones can differentiate several million different hues, but requires a higher light intensity of 10 to 10^6 cd/m². Taking advantage of this phenomenon, photopic imaging converts the original grey values **(Fig. 10.4a)** to color values **(Fig. 10.4b)**, based on the original histograms of the signals. This considerably improves the detection of details. However, it is not sufficient to add synthetic color to the monitor image. Instead, the real-time display of a faithful color-coded image requires extensive computations. An additional advantage of this technique is the ability to perform the examination with less darkening of the examination room.

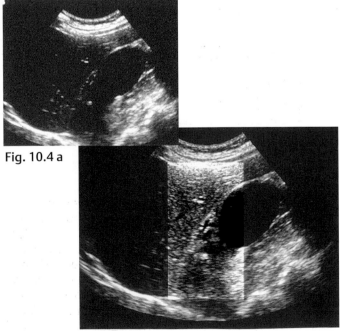

Fig. 10.4 a

Fig. 10.4 b

The material in the following six pages is not an absolute prerequisite for the first practice sessions and can be skipped. The novice may prefer to move directly from here to Session 1 (see page 17), but should return to these pages at a later time to reinforce the fundamental understanding of sonography.

Harmonic Imaging

This technique does not use the fundamental frequency of the transmitted sound waves, but their integer multiples, so-called harmonics or "harmonic frequencies" (e.g., 7.0 MHz for a fundamental 3.5 MHz). These harmonic overtones become more intense with increasing penetration, but their amplitude (intensity) remains markedly less than the fundamental signal. These harmonic frequencies have the advantage that they scarcely arise near the transducer, but

grow with increasing penetration **(Fig. 11.1)**. Consequently, they are not subjected to the major sources of scattered noise. Why do harmonic frequencies build up with increasing penetration?

Ultrasound waves become distorted when traversing tissues of changing acoustic properties. Their pressure waves compress and relax the tissue during their propagation. While compressed tissue increases the speed of sound, relaxed tissue lowers the speed with slower progression of the pressure wave. The wave form **(Fig. 11.2)** becomes distorted and induces harmonic waves. It is an accumulative process that expands with increasing penetration. Consequently, the amplitudes of the harmonic frequencies initially widen with increasing penetration until the expansion is offset by the general absorption **(Fig. 11.1)**.

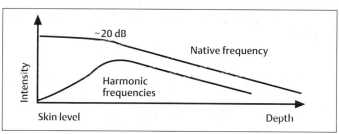

Fig. 11.1

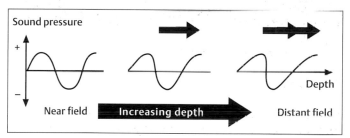

Fig. 11.2

Second Harmonic Imaging

This technique uses only the doubled frequency of the fundamental signal for imaging. To avoid an overlapping of the range of the harmonic frequency with the range of the fundamental frequency **(Fig. 11.3a)**, a narrow-band signal must be used to distinguish the strong components of the fundamental frequency from the weaker components of the

harmonic frequency **(Fig. 11.3b)**. The narrow bandwidth of the signal leads to a somewhat reduced contrast and spatial resolution. In spite of these shortcomings, this technique has markedly improved detection of details **(Fig. 11.4b)** compared to conventional sonography **(Fig. 11.4a)**, especially in obese patients (who have excessive scattering in the abdominal wall).

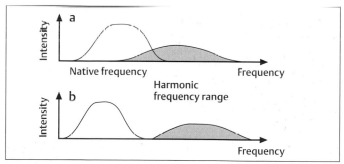

Fig. 11.3

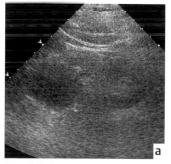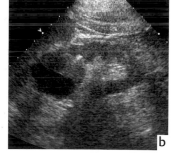

Fig. 11.4

Phase Inversion Technique

This is a recently introduced broadband technique that enables the dynamic optimization of harmonic multiples of the transmitted frequency with a broader bandwidth (Ensemble®THI) **(Fig. 12.1c)**. With this technique, the image optimization no longer depends on the narrow bandwidth of the fundamental frequency **(Fig. 12.1a)** for clean separation from its harmonic multiples **(Fig. 12.1b)**. Two subsequent pulses are transmitted in such a way that the phase (deviation of the pressure upward = positive and, respectively, downward = negative) of the second pulse is inverted to the phase of the first pulse **(Fig. 11.5)**.

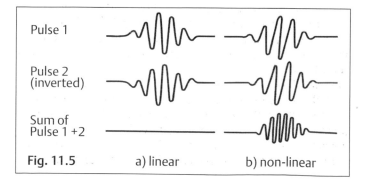

Fig. 11.5   a) linear   b) non-linear

If the echoes of both signals are added, the sum equals zero as long as the signal has not undergone any changes within the body. As a result, both fundamental frequency echoes are suppressed (**Fig. 11.5a**) and the second harmonic signal components are enhanced (**Fig. 11.5b**). **Figure 12.2** depicts a case showing acoustic shadowing (⬆ ⬆ ⬆) distal to intrarenal calcifications (**b**), which are undetectable by conventional imaging (**a**). In addition, the renal cyst (⬊) appears better demarcated and can be classified as benign with greater confidence.

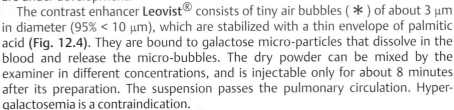

Native frequency   2nd harmonic imaging   Broadband harmonic imaging [MHz]

a   b   c

Fig. 12.1

Contrast Enhancement

The echogenicity of blood and tissue can be enhanced with tiny micro-bubbles with a diameter of 3 to 5 μm that pass through the capillaries and change the impedance within the bloodstream (**Fig. 12.3**). So far, three contrast enhancement agents have been introduced, and about 50 additional agents are under development.

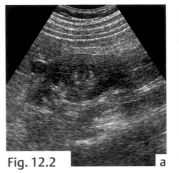

Fig. 12.2 　　　　　　　　　a 　　　　　　　b

The contrast enhancer **Leovist**® consists of tiny air bubbles (✱) of about 3 μm in diameter (95% < 10 μm), which are stabilized with a thin envelope of palmitic acid (**Fig. 12.4**). They are bound to galactose micro-particles that dissolve in the blood and release the micro-bubbles. The dry powder can be mixed by the examiner in different concentrations, and is injectable only for about 8 minutes after its preparation. The suspension passes the pulmonary circulation. Hypergalactosemia is a contraindication.

The contrast enhancer **Optison**® consists of octafluorpropan micro-bubbles with human serum albumin as adjunct and has been primarily applied in cardiology so far. The mean size of the microbubbles is 3.7 μm (shown in **Fig. 12.5** in comparison with erythrocytes). The octafluorpropan is almost completely eliminated by the lungs within about 10 minutes after its administration. Any possible virus contamination is inactivated by plasma fractionation with 40% alcohol and by pasteurization at 60 degrees centigrade (140 degrees Fahrenheit) for 10 hours.

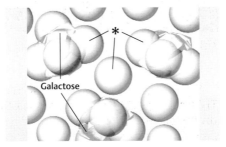

Fig. 12.3

The contrast enhancer **Sonovue**® consists of a watery solution of sulfur hexafluoride (SF_6), which is stabilized by a phospholipid layer (**Fig. 12.6**). The median size of the bubbles is about 2.5 μm (90% < 8 μm) with an osmolarity of 290 mOsmol/kg. This contrast enhancer has the advantage that its suspension is stable for 6 hours and can be used for several applications.

The best results are achieved in conjunction with tissue harmonic imaging (THI), referred to as **"contrast harmonic imaging (CHI)"**. A specific sound pressure excites the bubbles to vibrate and to emit an enhanced harmonic echo. As a result, CHI (**Fig. 12.7b**) can detect multiple hepatic metastases markedly better than unenhanced conventional images (**Fig. 12.7a**).

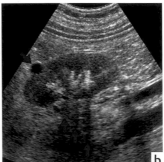

✱

Galactose

Fig. 12.4

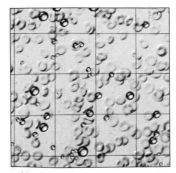

Fig. 12.5

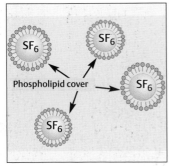

SF_6 　　　　SF_6

Phospholipid cover 　→ SF_6

SF_6

Fig. 12.6

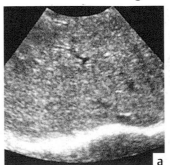

a 　　　　　　b

Fig. 12.7

Spatial Compounding (SonoCT®)

This is another technique to suppress artifacts. The "real-time compound imaging" does not scan the grid lines individually **(Fig. 13.1a)**, but at different angles with real-time computation of the image **(Fig. 13.1b)**. By adding up to nine sections, a precise display of the tissue information can be achieved, as illustrated by the morphology of an arteriosclerotic plaque **(Fig. 13.2a)** in comparison with conventional imaging **(Fig. 13.2b)**.

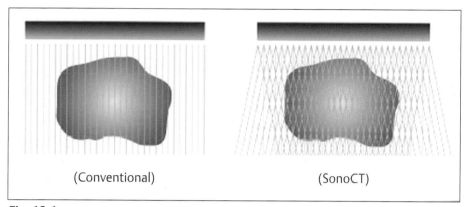

(Conventional)   (SonoCT)

Fig. 13.1

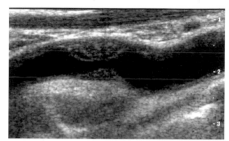

Fig. 13.2 a

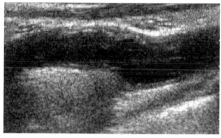

Fig. 13.2 b

Definite advantages have also been observed in sonography of the breast and musculoskeletal system: **Figure 13.3b** shows the improved visualization of an entire biopsy needle (↘) in the breast parenchyma in comparison with the conventional image **(Fig. 13.3a)**, enabling a more exact localization of the suspicious lesion.

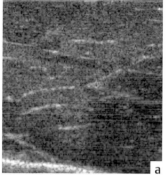

Fig. 13.3

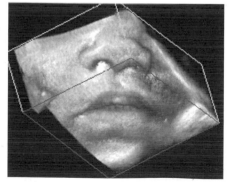

Fig. 13.4

Especially, the combination of SonoCT® scanning with THI (see page 11) has shown promising results with detailed display of hepatic lesions **(Fig. 13.5)** and fetal morphology in prenatal evaluation **(Fig. 13.6)**. The computer programs available today are capable of combining SieClear® or SonoCT® with three-dimensional visualization **(Fig. 13.7)** and with panoramic imaging **(Fig. 13.4)**, for instance, with visualization of almost the entire liver at the level of the hepatic venous system (see page 34).

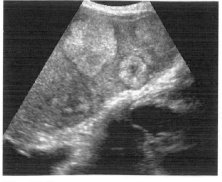

Fig. 13.5

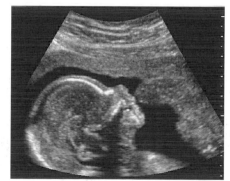

Fig. 13.6

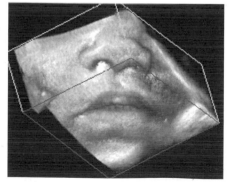

Fig. 13.7

Reverberation

The monitor image does not always reflect the true echogenicity. There are phenomena not corresponding to morphologic findings and referred to as "artifacts." The image generation illustrated on page 6 assumes that the echoes always return directly from the point of reflection straight to the transducer. The processing unit makes the same assumption when computing the depth of the site of reflection. In reality, this might not be a valid assumption.

On its way back to the transducer, the sound waves can be partially reflected at an encountered impedance change and sent back into the depth of the tissues, where they are again reflected to reach the transducer eventually but with some delay (**Fig. 14.1**). The delayed arrival of the returning echoes is incorrectly computed as increased depth, since the echoes are falsely assigned to a location further distal. In general, this phenomenon is lost in the background noise of the image, but it can project into anechoic areas, such as the lumen of the urinary bladder (**38**) or gallbladder, as lines parallel to the abdominal wall (**51a** in **Fig. 14.2**). These reverberation echoes can repeatedly occur in the abdominal wall, producing several lines parallel to each other (**51a**).

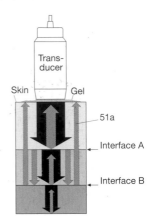

Fig. 14.1

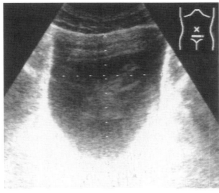

Fig. 14.2 a

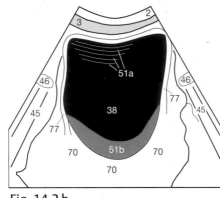

Fig. 14.2 b

Section Thickness Artifacts

An indistinctness of the wall of the urinary bladder can appear along the wall away from the transducer. If the wall of the urinary bladder (**77**), cyst or gallbladder is not perpendicular to the sound beam, the wall is indistinctly visualized and appears thickened (**51b** in **Fig. 14.2**). Such a section thickness artifact must be distinguished from layered material (small concrements, sludge, blood clots) (**52**) (**Fig. 14.3**), which usually is more distinctly demarcated from the remaining lumen and can be disturbed with the transducer.

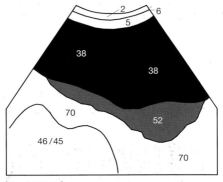

Fig. 14.3 a

Fig. 14.3 b

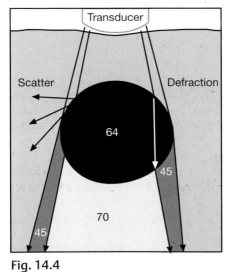

Fig. 14.4

(Distal) Acoustic Enhancement

Relative enhancement of the echoes (**70**) occurs distal to large vessels or cavities (**64**) filled with homogeneous (anechoic) fluid (**Fig. 14.4**). In **Figures 14.2** and **14.3**, this causes the tissue distal to the urinary bladder (**38**) to appear almost white and to become unsuitable for interpretation. How does this happen?

Wherever sound waves travel for some distance through homogeneous fluid, they encounter no reflections and attenuate less. This casts an echogenic (= bright) band (**70**) behind the gallbladder, urinary bladder, cysts or major vessels that does not correspond to the "true" characteristics of the underlying tissue. The acoustic enhancement, however, can serve as discriminating criterion, for instance, to differentiate an anechoic cyst (showing distal acoustic enhancement as it is above a certain size) from a hypoechoic hepatic lesion (generally lacking this phenomenon).

Acoustic Shadowing

Bands of markedly reduced echogenicity (hypoechoic or anechoic = black) are found behind strongly reflecting structures (ribs, calcium-containing stones, some ligaments, but also gastric or intestinal air). This can impair the visualization of soft-tissue structures beneath overlying ribs or the pubic symphysis as much as behind air-containing bowel loops or stomach. This effect, however, can be exploited to reveal calcific stones (49) in the gallbladder (14) as in **Figure 15.1**, renal stones (49) as in **Figure 54.2** and atherosclerotic plaques (49) as in **Figure 23.1**. Intestinal air can produce either hypoechoic (= dark) acoustic shadows or, through reverberations, a tapering tail of hyperechoic (= bright, "comet-tail") artifacts.

Edge shadows (45) can be created by round cavities tangentially hit by sound waves (**Fig. 15.2**). They are caused by scatter and refraction (**Fig. 14.4**). The case of a gallbladder (14)

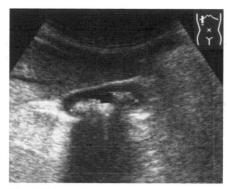

Fig. 15.1 a

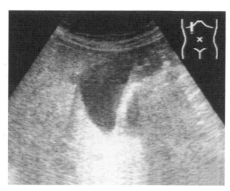

Fig. 15.2 a

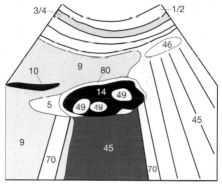

Fig. 15.1 b

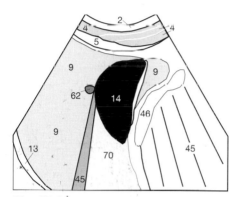

Fig. 15.2 b

with an edge shadow as shown in **Figure 15.2** requires careful analysis to avoid the edge shadow being falsely assigned to an acoustic shadow (45) from a focally spared area (62) in a fatty liver (9). Acoustic shadowing from duodenal air (46) is commonly mistaken for shadowing stones in the adjacent gallbladder (14). Do you remember the phenomenon that is responsible for the falsely echogenic visualization (70) of the hepatic parenchyma distal to the gallbladder (14) in **Figure 15.2**?

Mirror Effect

Strongly reflecting interfaces, such as the diaphragm (13), can deflect sound waves in such a way that they mimic a lesion on the other side of the reflecting surface, seen here as mirror artifact of the diaphragm (**Fig. 15.3**). The sound waves are deflected laterally by the diaphragm, hit a reflecting interface (R), bounce back to the diaphragm, and from there return to the transducer. Since the processing unit solely computes the distance of the object from the

time elapsed between emitting and recording of the sound pulse, the reflecting surface (R) is spuriously placed too deep (R') along the axis of the incident sound beam. **Figure 15.4** shows the inferior vena cava (16) as a mirror image projected above the diaphragm (16'). In addition, the mirror image of the hepatic parenchyma (9) is seen on the pulmonary side of the diaphragm (9'). Another example of a mirror artifact is found in **Figure 35.2**.

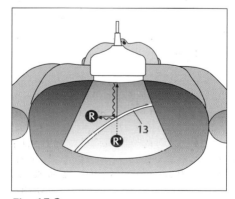

Fig. 15.3

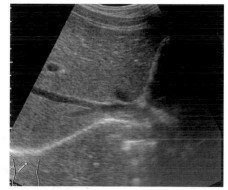

Fig. 15.4 a

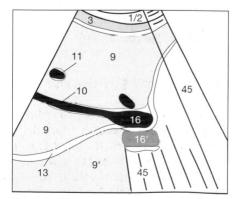

Fig. 15.4 b

Side Lobe Artifact

So far, we have assumed that sound waves exclusively propagate along the primary sound beam, which is directed from top to bottom on the sonographic image (dark blue lobe in **Fig. 16.1**). In reality, however, the transducer emits several so-called "secondary or side lobes" that can induce many scatter and blurring effects. If such a side lobe hits a strong reflecting surface, the obliquely deflected sound waves are shifted by the processing unit to a false adjacent location on the image display (**Fig. 16.2**). The more lateral the deflection of the sound waves, the longer their traveling time and the farther away the echoes are projected from their origin by the processing unit. This often leads to an arc-like extension of a strongly reflecting interface (✎ in **Fig. 16.3**).

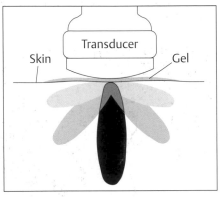

Fig. 16.1

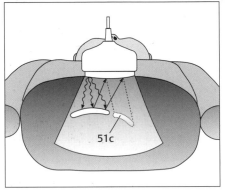

Fig. 16.2

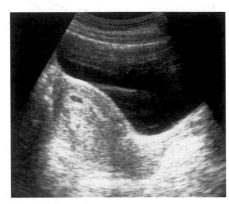

Fig. 16.3

Quiz for the Technical Fundamentals / Technique

Before any practical exercises with the ultrasound equipment and / or before Session 1, you are invited to test whether you have truly understood and can recall everything so far, and whether you still have knowledge gaps. You can check your answers by going back to the preceding pages. The answer to the image question no. 4 is on page 106.

1. Which structures are (almost) always anechoic = black on sonographic images? Name four physiologic and four pathologic findings.

Physiologic:	Pathologic:
-	-
-	-
-	-
-	-

2. Which frequencies are used for which clinical question and why? Name the respective bandwidth in MHz and sketch the monitor display of the corresponding type of transducer. When do you use which transducer? Explain why.

3. How does the processing unit compute the depth of the reflected echo? Can you deduce at least three artifacts from this principle and explain them to others?

4. Look at **Fig. 16.4** and explain the names and origin of all artifacts you can find.

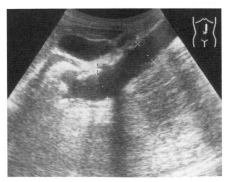

Fig. 16.4

Spatial Orientation

Before you begin with the practical orientation, even before any practical exercises in an ultrasound workshop, you should become familiar with the spatial orientation in the 3D-space of the abdomen. To make the first step easy, only two planes, which are perpendicular to each other, are initially considered: the vertical (= sagittal) image plane and the horizontal (= transverse) plane. It requires your active participation to have these planes mentally ingrained.

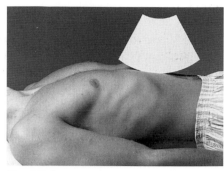

Fig. 17.1 a

Step 1: Take a coffee filter (you should find one in any hospital) or draw the shape of a coffee filter on a piece of paper. Its shape resembles a sonographic image generated by a convex transducer (see page 9).
Visualize along which border of the image you will find the anterior, posterior, left, right, superior and inferior structures of the patient, if you view the image plane according to the international convention, from the patient's right side **(Fig. 17.1a)**.

Hold the coffee filter to your abdomen and imagine sound waves that propagate from the midline of your abdomen toward the spine. Write down four of six offered directions at the borders of the filter or your drawing. Two are obviously wrong – and you should figure out why. (It is worth your while; you will remember this for good if you figure it out yourself.)

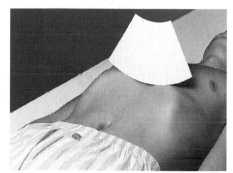

Fig. 17.1 b

Step 2: Before you look up the solution, repeat the same exercise for the axial (= transverse) section. For this section, however, the convention states that the image plane is placed on the monitor as seen from below (from the patient's feet) **(Fig. 17.1b)**. Write down four of the six adjectives on the back of the filter: two will be wrong again, but they will be different. OK. After you have reviewed your results, please check the solution on page 106.

The next problem addresses superimposed intestinal air and its corresponding acoustic shadowing. The solution usually is not more gel (as many beginners think), but in grading compression of the transducer.

How Much Pressure Do I Apply on the Transducer?

The beginner generally is too concerned about causing any discomfort to the patient and does not press the transducer strongly enough on the anterior abdominal wall. This reluctance (↓↓↓) leaves the air in stomach and intestines **(26)**, with acoustic shadowing **(45)** preventing the visualization of the posteriorly located pancreas **(33)** and adjacent vessels **(Fig. 17.2a)**. Furthermore, the extrahepatic common bile duct **(66)** and the portal vein **(11)** are frequently acoustically obscured by duodenal or gastric air.

For an adult patient, this can be solved by graded pressure (↓↓↓) on the transducer, beginning slowly to avoid startling the patient or causing any pain **(Fig. 17.3)**. The trick is to maintain a steady pressure: This will increasingly (and gently) push the intestinal air out of the field of view, making the interfering acoustic shadows **(45)** disappear so that the pancreas **(33)** and the other vessels become clearly visible **(Fig. 17.2b)**.

This approach is especially helpful for visualizing retroperitoneal lymph nodes and vessels, even in the mid-abdomen and lower abdomen. In infants, these maneuvers are usually superfluous or even counterproductive (because of their lower pain threshold and reactive resistance).

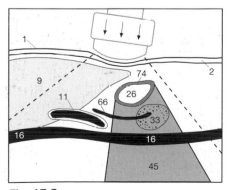

Fig. 17.2 a

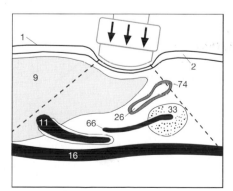

Fig. 17.2 b

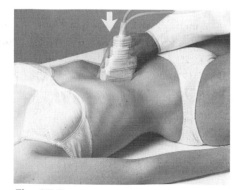

Fig. 17.3

Relevance of Adequate Breathing Instructions

Naturally, the novice is reluctant to give instructions directly to the patient. Regardless, almost all patients are very cooperative when it is explained to them that for an adequate image quality of the upper abdomen (and for the validity of the findings), it is crucial that the patient takes a deep breath to move the liver caudally. Why?

In the neutral breathing position (**Fig. 18.1a**), the liver and spleen are not the only structures superimposed by acoustic shadows. The pancreas (**33**) and its surroundings are often not seen because of gastric air (**26**). However, by moving the liver (**9**) lower (**→**) with maximum inspiration (**Fig. 18.1b**), gas-containing bowel loops and the stomach (**26**) are displaced inferiorly, opening the view of the pancreas and important nodal sites. Taking advantage of respiration-induced motion also makes it easier to visualize kidneys and porta hepatis (see below).

Please use clear breathing instructions, such as "take a deep breath with your mouth open (pause) and hold your breath." After an adequate breath-holding period (up to a maximum of 20 seconds) or immediately after a frozen image is obtained, the command to continue breathing should be given. This remark is not as trivial as you may think.

Good breathing instructions are not only well received by the patient, but also avoid any undue strain on the patient's respiratory condition and expedite the examination of the upper abdomen. Of course, these maneuvers are superfluous when examining the lower abdomen.

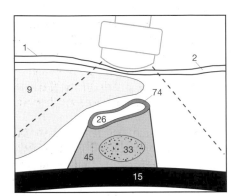

Fig. 18.1a

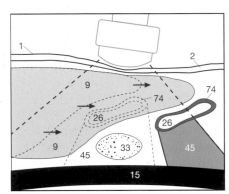

Fig. 18.1b

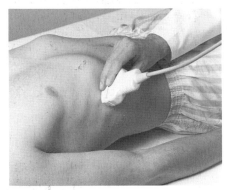

Fig. 18.2

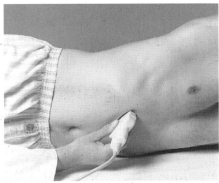

Fig. 18.3

Visualization of the Porta Hepatis

If the above-mentioned tricks fail to visualize the porta hepatis, try to visualize it in expiration through an intercostal space (**Fig. 18.2**). If this also is unsuccessful, turn the patient onto the left lateral decubitus position (**Fig. 18.3**). The liver's own weight moves it closer to the anterior abdominal wall, hopefully displacing interfering intestinal loops and opening a view of the porta hepatis including its important surrounding structures (compare page 30).

Check Your Combinatorial Ability: Look at **Figures 18.4** and **18.5**. Both images are of poor quality. Decide which image was obtained with too little gel and which with too little pressure. **Fig. 18.6** shows an image obtained under optimal conditions with sufficient pressure and an adequate amount of gel. All three images were obtained on the same patient in rapid succession. (The solution is found on page 106).

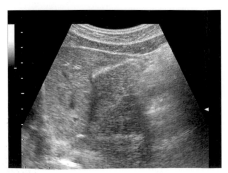

Fig. 18.4

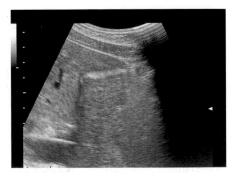

Fig. 18.5

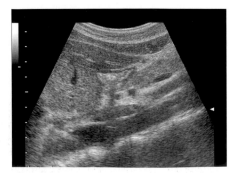

Fig. 18.6

Before you work on this page, please do the exercise on page 17 to familiarize yourself with spatial orientation from sagittal planes. You should proceed only after you have become comfortable with this kind of orientation and its physical principles (page 6-16), since this essential basic knowledge is assumed here.

The goal of scrutinizing the retroperitoneum is not limited to evaluating the retroperitoneal vessels to exclude, for instance, an abdominal aortic aneurysm or a thrombosis in the inferior vena cava. An additional goal is to become familiar with the orientation of the traversing vessels, since transversely or obliquely sectioned vessels are easily mistaken for ovoid lymph nodes (LN), which can appear hypoechoic. Furthermore, the correct identification of the individual vessels makes spatial orientation and correctly assigning other structures much easier. The **transducer** should be perpendicularly placed on the epigastric region along the linea alba and the sound beam swept through the upper abdomen in a fanlike fashion (**Fig. 19.1**). For the time being, it should suffice to memorize the normal sectional

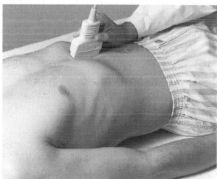

Fig. 19.1

anatomy. With the transducer tilted to the patient's right side (**Fig. 19.2a**), the aorta (**15**), celiac axis (**32**), and superior mesenteric artery (SMA) (**17**) are found to the left of the spine and posterior to the liver (**9**). On its left side, the image displays the thin hyperechoic curvilinear diaphragm (bare area) (**13**), which forms an hypoechoic muscular extension (**13a**) at the ventral margin of the aortic aperture. Just like the esophagus (**34**), it can be mistaken for a retroperitoneal lymph node. More inferiorly, the left renal vein (**25**) is sectioned transversely as it crosses between the superior mesenteric artery (SMA) (**17**) and the aorta (**15**). Because of its hypoechoic and ovoid appearance, it can be easily mistaken for a lymph node by the novice. Comparison with the transverse section at the same level (**Fig. 26.3**) and the anatomic diagram (**Fig 25.2**) clarifies this finding further. More anterior (closer to the transducer), the confluence (**12**) of the portal vein is found at the posterior border of the pancreas (**33**). Air in the gastric lumen (**26**) can cast interfering acoustic shadows at the inferior hepatic border.

Now tilt the transducer to the patient's left side (**Fig. 19.3a**) to visualize the inferior vena cava (IVC) (**16**) in the right paravertebral space and its continuation into the right atrium (**116**). The diameter of aorta and IVC are determined perpendicular to their longitudinal axes (see pages 21/23). Hepatic veins (**10**), branches of the left portal vein branch (**11**) and (anterior to it) branches of the hepatic artery (**18**) can be delineated within the liver (**9**). A thin echogenic septum separates the caudate lobe (**9a**) from the remaining hepatic parenchyma (**9**) in this plane. The caudate lobe should not measure more than 5.0 cm craniocaudally and 2.5 cm anteroposteriorly.

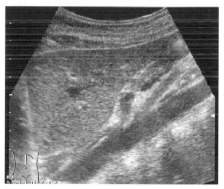

Fig. 19.2 a

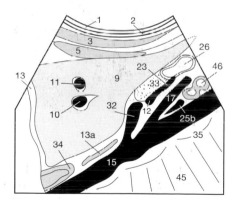

Fig. 19.2 b

Fig. 19.2 c

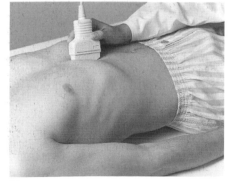

Fig. 19.3 a

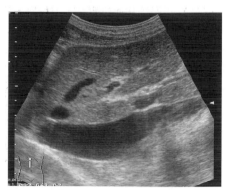

Fig. 19.3 b

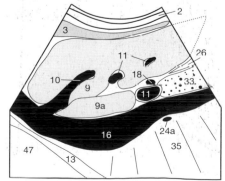

Fig. 19.3 c

After the upper retroperitoneum has been scrutinized, move the transducer inferiorly (➜) along the aorta (AO) and inferior vena cava (**Fig. 20.1a**). The evaluation should not be limited to the vascular lumina, but should include the spaces along the vessels by tilting the transducer from left to right to search for enlarged perivascular lymph nodes (**Fig. 19.1**), which are characteristically seen as ovoid hypoechoic space-occupying lesions (see pages 22 and 29). Pathologically enlarged lymph nodes can also be encountered anterior or posterior to the large vessels as well as in the aortocaval space.

In the absence of any retroaortic space-occupying process, the distance between the posterior aortic wall and the anterior vertebral borders should not exceed 5 mm. Preferably, these measurements should be obtained in two planes (see pages 25 and 26).

Distal to the aortic bifurcation, the branching iliac vessels are delineated and evaluated in the same way by sweeping the sound beam parallel (**Fig. 20.1b**) and perpendicular (**Fig. 20.1c**) to the longitudinal vascular axis.

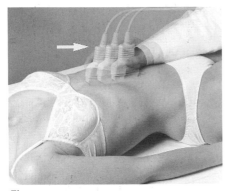

Fig. 20.1 a

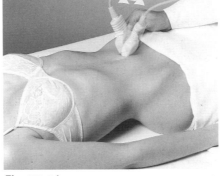

Fig. 20.1 b

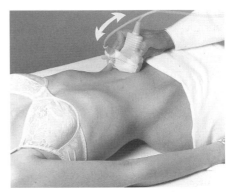

Fig. 20.1 c

The confluence of external (**22a**) and internal (**22b**) iliac veins is another preferential site for regional nodal enlargement (**Fig. 20.2**). The iliac artery (**21**) is anterior (i.e., upper aspect of the image) to the vein. The compression test can clarify inconclusive findings. Because of their low intraluminal pressure, veins are more easily compressible than arteries.

On transverse section (**Fig. 20.3**), the iliac vessels can be easily distinguished from hypoechoic fluid-filled intestinal loops (**46**) by the intestinal peristaltic activities. If necessary, one can try to trigger the peristaltic waves by rapid alteration of the applied pressure on the transducer.

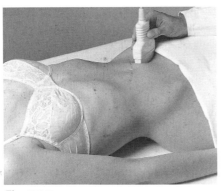

Fig. 20.2 a

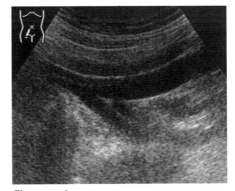

Fig. 20.2 b

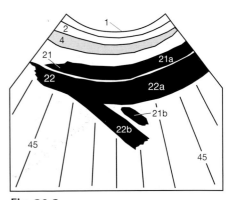

Fig. 20.2 c

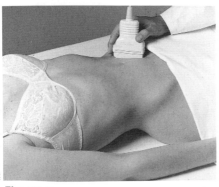

Fig. 20.3 a

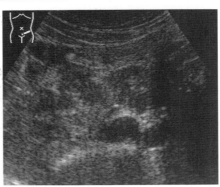

Fig. 20.3 b

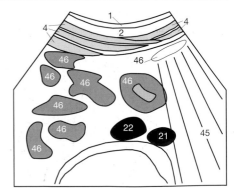

Fig. 20.3 c

Localized dilations of the vascular lumen are mostly caused by atherosclerotic lesions and local weakening of the arterial wall. It rarely is post-traumatic. A dilation of the aorta exceeding 25 mm to 30 mm is referred to as an ectasia, and this can be found in addition to an aneurysm **(Fig. 21.1)**, which is defined in the abdomen as a suprarenal diameter of more than 30 mm (the upper limit for the aortic arch is 40 mm).

The dilation can be fusiform or saccular. It can be complicated by dissection of the arterial wall (dissecting aneurysm) or by circumferential intraluminal clot formation **(52)** with possible peripheral or abdominal emboli. Risk factors for a rupture are increasing diameter of the aneurysm, a diameter exceeding 50 mm or 60 mm, or an eccentric diverticulum-like bulging of the aortic wall. For a thrombosed aneurysm, a concentric lumen can be protective while an eccentric lumen increases the risk for rupture. As a general rule, the risk of a rupture increases with the size of the aneurysm, but the surgical indication depends on many individual factors and no absolute threshold can be defined.

If an aneurysm is detected, the sonographic examination should report its maximal length **(Fig. 21.2)** and diameter **(Fig. 21.3)** as well as any detected dissection or thrombi and possible involvement of any visceral branches (celiac axis, SMA, and renal and iliac arteries).

The main arterial supply of the spinal cord (Adamkiewicz artery) has a variable segmental level and usually defies sonographic visualization because of its small lumen. In these cases, supplementary spiral CT or invasive DSA are needed to determine the arterial supply of the spinal cord.

Checklist for Aortic Aneurysm

Suprarenal aorta: < 25 mm (normal)
Aortic ectasia: 25-30 mm
Aneurysm: > 30 mm
Signs of increased rupture risk:
- Progressing dilation
- Diameter > 60 mm
- Diverticular rather than fusiform
- Evidence of dissection
- Eccentric lumen

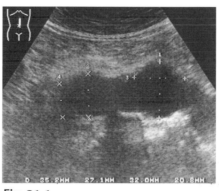

Fig. 21.1 a

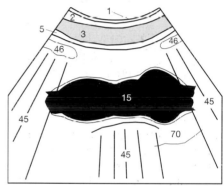

Fig. 21.1 b

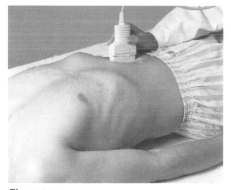

Fig. 21.2 a

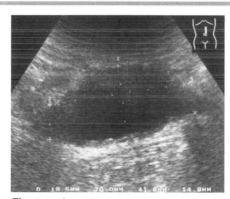

Fig. 21.2 b

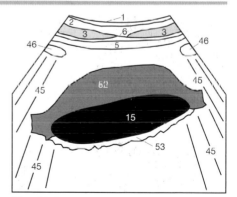

Fig. 21.2 c

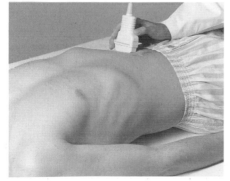

Fig. 21.3 a

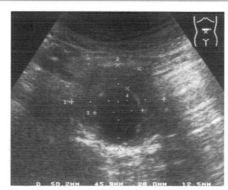

Fig. 21.3 b

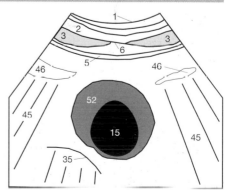

Fig. 21.3 c

Lymph nodes (LN) **(55)** are generally delineated as hypoechoic ovoid structures. Above all, they must be differentiated from axially or obliquely sectioned blood vessels, which can fulfil the same criteria on the static images. Therefore, we recommend scrutinizing each region dynamically in two planes by continuously tilting the transducer. Using this approach, vessels either widen (and join other vessels) or taper, while lymph nodes appear and disappear abruptly. An unsystematic approach to lymph nodes forgoes this opportunity to discriminate.

In the lower abdomen, axially sectioned bowel loops with hypoechoic content and absent peristalsis can resemble lymph nodes. Thrombosed veins are another diagnostic possibility. In addition to an enlargement of lymph nodes secondary to reactive inflammatory changes and metastatic deposits, nodal enlargement is primarily found with malignant lymphoma (Hodgkin disease or non-Hodgkin lymphoma).

Diagnostic Assignment of Enlarged Lymph Nodes

The normal size of the abdominal lymph nodes is stated to be 7-10 mm along their long axis. Larger and still normal lymph nodes of up to 20 mm in longitudinal diameter can be found in the inguinal region and along the distal external iliac artery **(Fig. 22.3)**. Normal and reactive inflammatory lymph nodes typically exhibit an ovoid configuration, with the longitudinal diameter divided by the transverse (the L/T ratio) greater than 2. This means that the length of a lymph node is more than twice its width when the transducer is placed along the longitudinal axis. Another sign of benign disease is the "hilar sign," which refers to an hyperechoic hilar structure in the center of the enlarged lymph node surrounded by a hypoechoic periphery. Inflammatory lymph nodes along the hepatoduodenal ligament **(Fig. 31.3)** often accompany viral hepatitis, cholecystitis/cholangitis or pancreatitis **(Fig. 27.3)**.

In contrast, round lymph nodes (L/T ratio of about 1.0) without a hilar sign suggest a pathologic change, whereby lymphomatous nodes generally are more markedly hypoechogenic than inflammatory or metastatic lymph nodes. The perfusion pattern of the color-coded duplex sonography within the lymph node provides additional information (please refer to the booklet "Teaching Manual of Color Duplex Sonography", listed at the end of the book).

Important for all enlarged lymph nodes are follow-up examinations to check for progression, central liquefaction (anechoic center in case of abscess formation) or regression; for instance after chemotherapy of the underlying disease. Furthermore, any possible hepatomegaly or splenomegaly should be documented and quantified.

The site of the primary tumor can be inferred from the known lymphatic pathways. In young men, for instance, para-aortic lymphadenopathy at the level of the kidneys suggests a testicular tumor.

Malignant lymphomas indent or displace adjacent vessels **(Fig. 22.2)**, but respect vascular walls and do not invade adjacent organs (see also page 29). Predominant involvement of the mesenteric lymph nodes **(55)** **(Figs. 22.1 and 22.2)** speaks for a non-Hodgkin lymphoma and against Hodgkin disease, which has a predilection for thoracic and retroperitoneal lymph nodes.

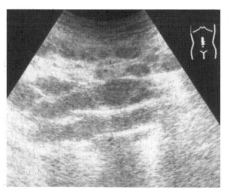

Fig. 22.1 a

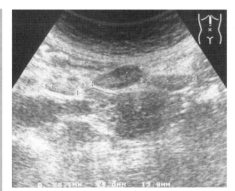

Fig. 22.1 b

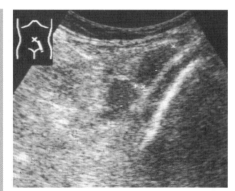

Fig. 22.2 a

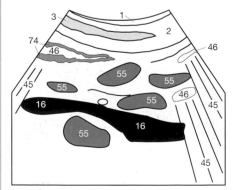

Fig. 22.2 b

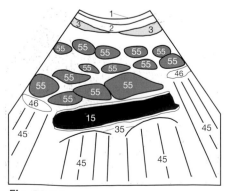

Fig. 22.3 a

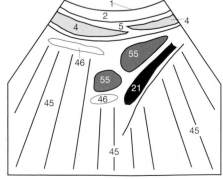

Fig. 22.3 b

The systematic evaluation of the retroperitoneum should delineate and document all abnormalities of the major vessels, as well as any changes of the aorta and the lymph nodes. The inferior vena cava can be distinguished from the aorta by its anatomic location (paravertebrally on the right instead of left) and also by the typical precordial double pulsation (instead of the single pulse of the aorta). Furthermore, atherosclerotic plaques **(49)** are frequent in older patients along the aortic wall **(15)**. If calcified, they are hyperechoic with acoustic shadowing **(45)**.

Right Heart Decompensation

The inferior vena cava **(16)** should be evaluated for a dilation exceeding 20 mm (or 25 mm in young athletes), which would suggest a venous congestion as manifestation of a right cardiac decompensation **(Fig. 23.2)**. The measurements are obtained perpendicular to the longitudinal vascular axis (!) and should not accidentally encompass the hepatic veins **(10)**, which enter the inferior vena cava subdiaphragmatically **(Fig. 23.2)**. In questionable cases, the "test of the collapsed IVC during forced inspiration" should be performed. The luminal diameter of the inferior vena cava is observed during forced maximal inspiration by asking the patient to take a deep breath with the mouth closed. The transmitted sudden drop in intrapleural pressure briefly collapses the subdiaphragmatic portion of the normal inferior vena cava, with its lumen reduced to a third or less of its initial value during quiet respiration.

It can be a challenge for the examiner to keep the sonographic section at the same level of the inferior vena cava during the respiratory movement of the thorax. Alternatively, this maneuver can be performed by observing a transverse image of the upper abdomen, or the luminal diameter of the hepatic veins can be assessed in the right subcostal oblique section (see page 34).

Do you remember why in **Figure 23.2**, the hepatic parenchyma appears more hyperechoic dorsal to the distended inferior vena cava than anterior to it? If not, return to page 9 and name this phenomenon.

Following an inguinal vascular puncture, the visualized distal iliac vessels **(Fig. 23.3)** can occasionally develop a hematoma **(50)** adjacent to the iliac artery **(21)** or vein **(22)**. If blood flows into this perivascular space through a persistent connection with the arterial lumen, a false (spurious) aneurysm is present, which differs from a true aneurysm in that the arterial layers are not stretched but torn with a resultant perivascular hematoma **(Fig. 23.3)**. Old inguinal hematomas must be differentiated from psoas abscesses and synovial cysts arising from the hip joint, and, when extending into the lower pelvis, from lymphoceles, large ovarian cysts and metastatic lymph nodes with central necrosis **(57)**.

Checklist for Right Heart Decompensation
- Dilated IVC > 20 mm or
  > 25 mm in young athletes
- Dilated hepatic veins > 6 mm (in the periphery)
- No collapsed IVC during forced inspiration
- Possible pleural effusion,
  initially often unilateral on the right

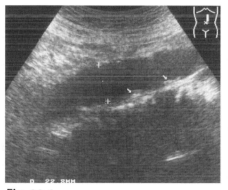

Fig. 23.1 a

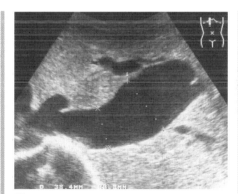

Fig. 23.2 a

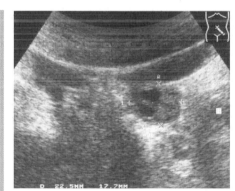

Fig. 23.3 a

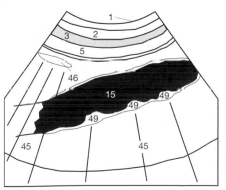

Fig. 23.1 b

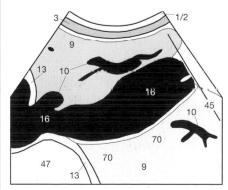

Fig. 23.2 b

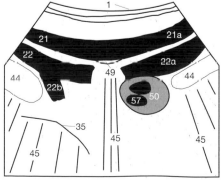

Fig. 23.3 b

Before proceeding to the material of Lesson 2, you should answer the following questions to test whether you have mastered the goal and contents of this first lesson. This quiz for self-assessment – if used in the spirit of self-improvement – can be quite effective to discourage superficial browsing through this workbook and to increase retention of the studied material, for the reader's long-term benefit. Enjoy the test.

The answers to questions 1 to 6 can be found on the preceding pages. The answers to the image question 7 can be looked up on page 107, of course only after the individual questions listed in the text have been addressed.

1. Which anatomic location corresponds to the left side of the sagittal sections? For practice, mark once again on the cone-shaped coffee filter shown here and review which of the following six spatial identifications cannot be found along the four borders: anterior, posterior, left, right, superior, inferior.

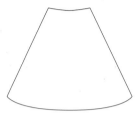

2. What is the maximal luminal diameter of the inferior vena cava and abdominal aorta? What is the definition of aortic ectasia and aortic aneurysm? Which clinical questions would you address sonographically when you find an aortic aneurysm? What are the limitations of sonography (better complementary examination with CT/DSA)?

AO suprarenal	<	mm	AO infrarenal	<	mm
IVC (athlete)	<	mm	AO ectasia	~	mm
AO aneurysm	>	mm			

3. Which three physiologic structures can mimic hypoechoic lymph nodes on the sagittal visualization of the aorta in the upper abdomen? Name all three and mark their positions in the standard planes by memory.

a) _____

b) _____

c) _____

4. Which two examinations can be added to exclude quickly a clinically suspected right heart decompensation in a case of a borderline luminal diameter of the inferior vena cava (without EKG)?

a) _____

b) _____

5. What maximum longitudinal diameter of retroperitoneal lymph nodes can still be called normal? Name the disease-specific criteria and normal findings of lymph nodes. What is the value of follow-up examinations for the evaluation of pathologically enlarged lymph nodes?

6. Look at the three transducers shown here **(Fig. 24.1)**. For each, write its name above and note its typical frequency range and applications below. Can you justify your decision?

7. Review this quiz image step by step. What is the image plane? Which organs and vessels are shown? Name as many structures as possible. How does this differ from an image with a normal finding? Try to provide a differential diagnosis.

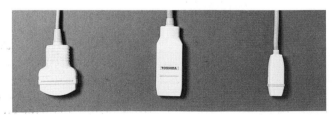

Fig. 24.1

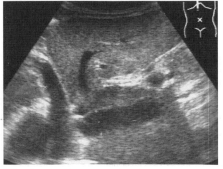

Fig. 24.2

Before working through the following pages, you should again review the sonographic sections obtained in the transverse plane. Where is the liver on a correctly oriented sonographic transverse section? Right or left? If you cannot answer this with confidence, you should consult page 17 and review the relative anatomic location of the organs as seen on transverse images by means of the coffee filter cone (the solution is found on page 106).

Aside from the pancreas, the perivascular lymph nodes are to be assessed. The transducer is rotated 90° counterclockwise and transversely placed on the upper abdomen. With the patient taking a deep breath and holding, the upper abdomen is systematically reviewed in craniocaudal direction while the transducer is rocked slowly and steadily (Fig. 25.1). In this manner, vessels can be easily identified by following their uninterrupted course and better differentiated from focal mass lesions.

On these transverse sections, the examiner is confronted with a multitude of arteries, veins,

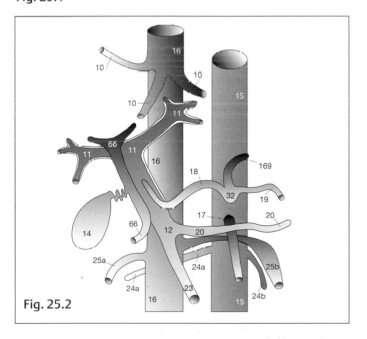

Fig. 25.1

biliary ducts and lymph nodes, all confined to a small space and to be differentiated from each other (all vessels are hypoechoic, but so are lymph nodes).

Do you remember where the left renal vein crosses to the contralateral right side, or whether the right renal artery traverses anterior or posterior to the right kidney? Refresh your basic anatomic knowledge by writing the names of all numbered structures in **Figure 25.2** on a separate sheet and adding the number codes below, initially without the help of the legend or an anatomy book. Though this approach might first appear somewhat cumbersome, it guarantees a considerably higher retention rate than simple recapitulation of an already annotated drawing. Then you unfold the back cover flap to compare your list with the legends and make correction if necessary. In the spirit of self-improvement, you should repeat this exercise on separate sheets until you can correctly assign all structures in **Figures 25.2** and **25.3**. Only then should you proceed to the subsequent pages, since both the concept of this workbook and the practical exercises adapted for this sonography course absolutely require familiarity with this basic knowledge.

Figure 25.3 primarily illustrates once again the topographic relationship of pancreas, duodenum and spleen to the most relevant vessels in the upper abdomen. For taking in the material, the three most important transverse sections of the upper abdomen are described and illustrated on the next page.

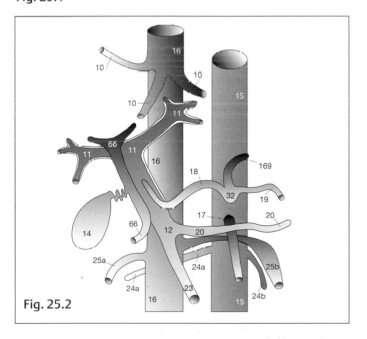

Fig. 25.2

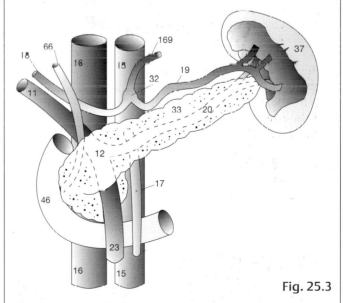

Fig. 25.3

Please complete this list with the help of both figures. Which number corresponds to which anatomic structure?

10 = _____

11 = _____

12 = _____

14 = _____

15 = _____

16 = _____

17 = _____

18 = _____

19 = _____

20 = _____

23 = _____

24 a = _____

24 b = _____

25a = _____

25b = _____

32 = _____

33 = _____

37 = _____

46 = _____

66 = _____

169 = _____

First, as a rule the patient must take a deep breath and hold it, so that the liver is moved inferiorly and a better acoustic window is created for the pancreas, lesser sac and origin of the major vessels (see page 18).

The hyperechoic skin (1), hypoechoic subcutaneous fatty tissue (2), and both rectus muscles (3) are directly beneath the transducer. A more cranial transverse section (Fig. 26.1) visualizes the celiac axis (32) together with the hepatic (18) and splenic (19) arteries. Its shape often resembles a whale fluke.

More inferiorly (Figs. 26.2 and 26.3), the rhomboid extension of the ligamentum teres (7) with its obliterated umbilical vein is delineated posterior to the linea alba (6). The lesser sac is seen as small cleft behind the liver (9) and, farther posterior to it, the pancreas (33). The tail of the pancreas is often obscured by air shadowing (45) arising from the stomach (26). The splenic vein (20) invariably runs directly along the posterior border of the pancreas. The left renal vein (25) is even more posterior between the superior mesenteric artery (17) and aorta (15), but runs more inferior (Fig. 26.3). Between both levels, the AMS (17) arises from the aorta. Occasionally, an atypical origin of the hepatic artery can be found here. Usually, the origin of the superior mesenteric artery is immediately below the origin of the celiac axis, as clearly illustrated on the sagittal images (Fig. 19.2).

It should be noted that the display inverts the position of the organs. The inferior vena cava (16), seen as an ovoid structure, is on the left side of the image, and the aorta (15), seen as a round structure, is on the right side anterior to the spine (35). The head of the pancreas characteristically surrounds the confluence (12) of the portal vein (11), which in the region of the lesser omentum is frequently obscured by duodenal air (46).

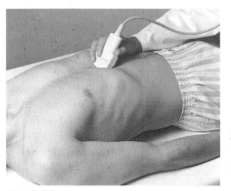

Fig. 26.1 a

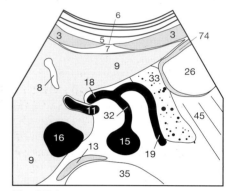

Fig. 26.1 b

Fig. 26.1 c

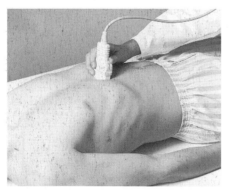

Fig. 26.2 a

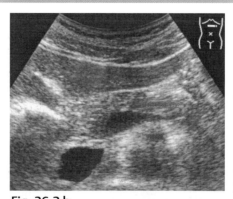

Fig. 26.2 b

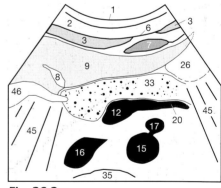

Fig. 26.2 c

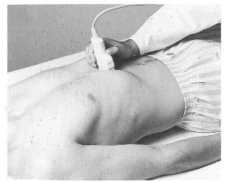

Fig. 26.3 a

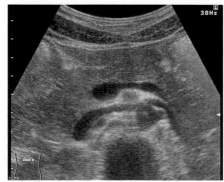

Fig. 26.3 b

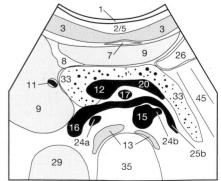

Fig. 26.3 c

Age-related Echogenicity

The echogenicity of the pancreas changes with increasing age. In young and slim patients, the parenchyma is hypoechoic, similar to the hepatic parenchyma. In older or obese patients (**Fig. 28.1a**), the impedance jumps increase in a progressively more heterogenous pancreatic parenchyma, leading to a hyperechoic (brighter) appearance of the pancreas.

The normal anteroposterior diameters of the pancreas are somewhat variable and should be < 3 cm for the head, < 2.0 cm for the body and < 2.5 cm for the tail. Frequent causes of pancreatitis include biliary obstruction (cholestasis) secondary to a stone lodged in the distal common bile duct (biliary pancreatitis), increased viscosity of the bile secondary to parenteral nutrition and, above all, alcoholism (alcohol-induced pancreatitis), which is, among other mechanisms, related to protein plugs obstructing the small pancreatic ducts.

Acute Pancreatitis

Acute pancreatitis of the first degree can initially lack any sonographic changes. The edema found in more advanced stages causes marked hypoechogenicity, possibly with an indistinct outline of the pancreas (**33**). The real contribution of sonography is not the early diagnosis of acute pancreatitis. This can be achieved better by laboratory tests or computerized tomography, in particular, in view of the pain and markedly increased bowel gas encountered with an acutely inflamed pancreas, which often interferes with sonographic imaging.

Chronic Pancreatitis

Chronic pancreatitis is characterized by heterogeneous fibrosis (**Fig. 27.1**), calcific deposits (**53**) and an undulated, irregularly outlined pancreas (**Figs. 27.1 and 27.2**). Moreover, a beaded or irregular dilation of the pancreatic duct (**75**) can occur (**Fig.27.2**). The normal pancreatic duct is smoothly outlined and measures 1 mm to up to 2 mm in diameter. Inflammatory lymph nodes (**55**) in the vicinity of the pancreas, for instance anterior to the portal vein (**11**), can accompany a pancreatitis (**Fig. 27.3**).

The role of sonography is the exclusion of other diagnostic possibilities, such as cholecystitis, choledocholithiasis and aortic aneurysm, and following the course of the disease. Furthermore, sonography can be used to detect secondary complications, such as thrombophlebitis of the adjacent splenic vein (**20**), possibly necessitating an additional color Doppler duplex sonography. Sonography can also visualize inflammatory infiltration of the neighboring duodenal or gastric wall (**46**, **26**) and pseudocysts. Moreover, necrotic paths in the retroperitoneum (grade II acute pancreatitis) should be discovered early, to proceed to surgical intervention or aspiration under sonographic or CT guidance if indicated.

The inflammation does not always involve the entire pancreas. Segmental or "groove" pancreatitis confined to certain segments of the organ also can occur. These manifestations cannot always be reliably differentiated from other localized space-occupying processes, such as a carcinoma.

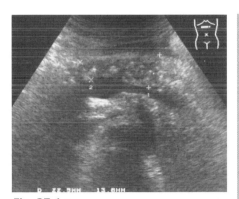

Fig. 27.1 a

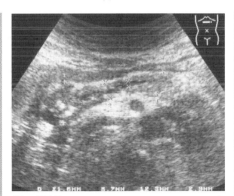

Fig. 27.2 a

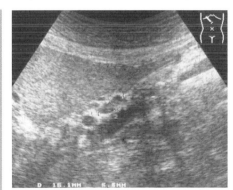

Fig. 27.3 a

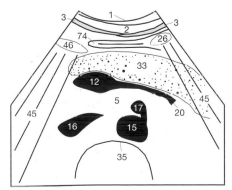

Fig. 27.1 b

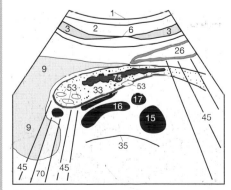

Fig. 27.2 b

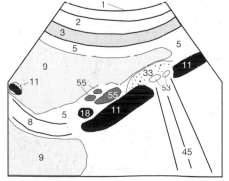

Fig. 27.3 b

Looking at the normal echogenicity of the pancreas (33) in **Figures 19.2** or **26.3** reveals no appreciable difference in comparison with the echogenicity of the liver. Increasing age or obesity uniformly increases the echogenicity due to pancreatic lipomatosis (**Fig. 28.1**). This accentuates the contrast to the anechoic splenic vein (20) and the portosplenic confluence (12).

Tumors of the pancreas (54) are generally more hypoechoic than the remaining pancreas and occasionally are barely discerned from adjacent bowel loops (peristalsis?) or peripancreatic lymph nodes. Pancreatic carcinomas have a poor prognosis and, depending on their location, remain clinically silent for a long time and often are detected late. The diagnosis is often made after compression of the common bile duct with resultant cholestasis or after an otherwise unexplained weight loss. Early retroperitoneal extension, nodal or hepatic metastases, and/or peritoneal

carcinomatosis are responsible for the poor five-year survival, which is below 10%.

Endocrine pancreatic tumors are generally small at the time of diagnosis because of their systemic hormonal effects and, as with all small pancreatic tumors, are best visualized by endosonography (**Fig. 28.3**). An annular transducer at the tip of an endoscope is positioned into the stomach or through the pylorus into the duodenum, surrounded by a water-filled balloon for acoustic coupling with the gastric or duodenal wall.

Because of the short penetration needed to reach the target structure, a high frequency (5.0-10.0 MHz) transducer can be selected, with corresponding higher resolution.

It should be kept in mind that the tail of the pancreas is best delineated by slightly rotating the transducer counterclockwise out of the transverse section (**Fig. 28.4**).

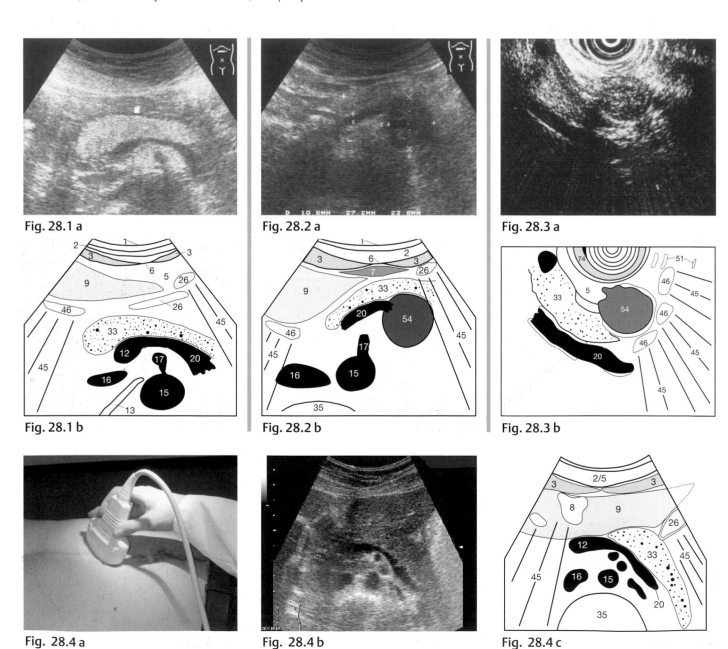

Fig. 28.1 a

Fig. 28.2 a

Fig. 28.3 a

Fig. 28.1 b

Fig. 28.2 b

Fig. 28.3 b

Fig. 28.4 a

Fig. 28.4 b

Fig. 28.4 c

Do you remember the criteria for distinguishing reactively enlarged inflammatory lymph nodes from lymphomatous lymph nodes and nodal metastases from other primary tumors? If not, please go back to page 22 and review the differential-diagnostic possibilities discussed there.

Especially under conditions poor for insonation (as in very obese patients), physiologic upper abdominal vessels (15, 16) should be definitively distinguished from pathologic lymph nodes (55) on transverse or oblique sections (Figs. 29.1 and 29.2). Familiarity with the normal vascular anatomy is therefore fundamental. Markedly hypoechoic lymph nodes that lack a more echogenic hilus and displace but do not invade adjacent veins are suggestive of a lymphoma, such as a chronic lymphatic leukemia (Fig. 29.2) (if this repetition bores you, one of the goals of learning has already been achieved...).

The pathologic lymph node (LN) shown in Figure 29.2 is situated directly anterior to and to the right of the bifurcation of the celiac axis (32) into common hepatic (18) and splenic artery (19). The resultant space-occupying effect obliterates the characteristic fluke-like configuration of the celiac axis. The cluster of enlarged lymph nodes (55) seen in Figure 29.1 elevates the hepatic artery (18) so far anteriorly that it follows an atypical elongated and straightened course where it arises from the celiac axis.

Occasionally, large nodal aggregates can be seen around and "encasing" the retroperitoneal or mesenteric vessels. In such cases, representative lymph nodes are identified and measured to address the question of interval growth on subsequent studies.

It is a good policy to measure the size of the liver and spleen whenever intra-abdominal or retroperitoneal lymph nodes are encountered. Furthermore, both organs must be carefully searched for heterogeneous infiltrations. Harmonic imaging techniques together with contrast-enhancing agents (see page 12) can be helpful in such cases (Fig. 12.8).

Without these methods, diffuse lymphomatous involvement of the splenic parenchyma does not always translate into sonographic changes. The infiltrated spleen can appear normal or may only show diffuse enlargement (Fig. 70.1).

Additional lymphadenopathy must be searched for in the inguinal, axillary and cervical regions. Paralytic fluid-filled intestinal loops are rarely mistaken for lymph nodes. An intestinal diverticulum (54) can mimic a tumor or enlarged lymph node (Fig 29.3). Occasionally, peristaltic activity elicited from a paralytic intestinal loop by graded compression of the transducer can instantaneously clarify the differential diagnosis.

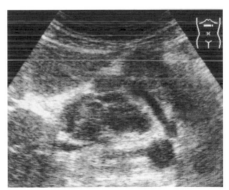

Fig. 29.1 a

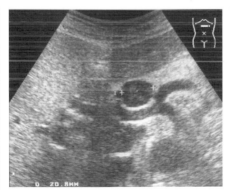

Fig. 29.2 a

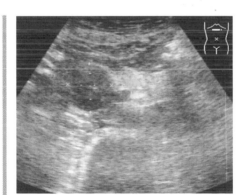

Fig. 29.3 a

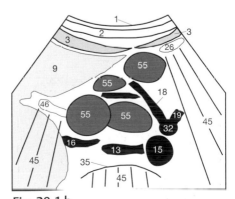

Fig. 29.1 b

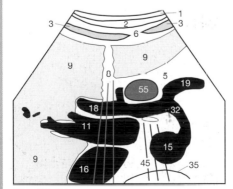

Fig. 29.2 b

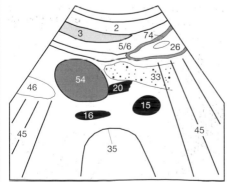

Fig. 29.3 b

To obtain the standard plane for the porta hepatis, we leave the transverse plane by rotating the transducer several degrees clockwise from the transverse orientation until the sound beam is parallel to the portal vein and parallel to left costal arch (Fig. 30.1a). Sometimes, the transducer has to be angled upward (Fig. 30.1b) to follow the course of the portal vein (11) from the porta hepatis to the confluence of splenic and superior mesenteric veins (12) (Fig. 30.2b). Visualizing the porta hepatis succeeds best by asking the patient to take a deep breath (don't forget breath commands!) so that the liver and porta hepatis move inferiorly from under the acoustic shadow of the ribs and lung.

Three hypoechoic structures can be delineated in the porta hepatis. The normal position of the portal vein (11) is immediately anterior to the obliquely sectioned (and expectedly ovoid) inferior vena cava (16). The common bile duct (66) and hepatic artery proper (18) are situated more anterior and seen just above the portal vein. The hepatic artery and its branches are segmentally visualized because of their undulating course, with the visualized segments appearing as round or ovoid structures (Fig. 30.2b) that should not be mistaken for periportal lymph nodes.

The common bile duct can be so narrow that it might be barely visible along the adjacent artery. Its normal diameter should be less than 6 mm. After cholecystectomy, it assumes somewhat of a reservoir function and can dilate up to 9 mm without pathologic significance. A borderline dilated common bile duct, e.g., obstruction caused by a stone, can no longer unmistakably be differentiated from adjacent vessels.

In this situation, the entire length of all three tubular structures must be systematically visualized to find their origin and, with it their identity. The hepatic artery is followed to the celiac axis, the portal vein to the portosplenic confluence or the splenic vein and the common bile duct to the pancreatic head. When visualizing the common bile duct, intraductal stones can be identified or excluded (see page 42). Alternatively or additionally, color Doppler duplex sonography, if available, can be used to differentiate these tubular structures.

The normal luminal width of the portal vein (11) is less than 13 mm when measuring the main branch perpendicular to its longitudinal axis. Dilation should only be suspected with measurements exceeding 15 mm. Measurements in between fall into the "gray zone" of physiologic variations. A dilated portal vein alone is an unreliable criterion for portal hypertension. The positive demonstration of portocaval collateral circulation is more accurate. The porta hepatis has to be systematically scrutinized to detect atypical periportal vascular convolutes (see page 31).

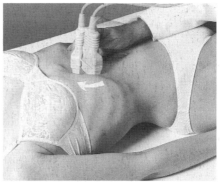

Fig. 30.1 a

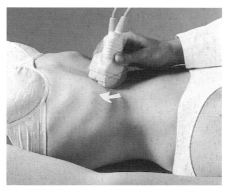

Fig. 30.1 b

Normal values:

Portal vein: < 13 mm
(maximum 15 mm)

Common bile duct   < 6 mm
(< 9 mm S / P cholecystectomy)

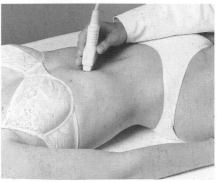

Fig. 30.2 a

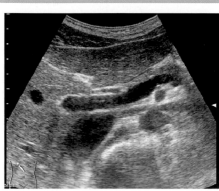

Fig. 30.2 b

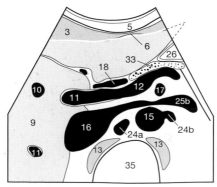

Fig. 30.2 c

The most common cause of increased pressure in the portal vein is impaired drainage secondary to cirrhosis. A direct compression of the portal vein by an adjacent tumor is found less frequently. A pancreatic tumor can involve the splenic vein or superior mesenteric vein, without affecting the portal vein. A dilated portal vein (11) should be considered suspicious for portal hypertension (Fig. 31.1) only if it exceeds 15 mm in diameter. The portal vein is measured perpendicular to the vessel's longitudinal axis, which usually is obliquely oriented on the sonographic image. The measurement should exclude the vascular wall.

It should be kept in mind that a splenomegaly of other etiology can dilate the splenic vein to more than 12 mm or the portal vein to more than 15 mm, without portal hypertension.

A dilated portal vein with a diameter of more than 13 mm is by itself an unreliable criterion for portal hypertension. Additional criteria are splenomegaly (Fig. 70.2), ascites (see pages 39, 58, 67) and, above all, portocaval collaterals at the porta hepatis. They usually drain congested blood from the portal system via a dilated coronary vein of the stomach and a dilated esophageal venous complex into the (hemi-)azygos vein, and from there into the superior vena cava. This can lead to the clinical complication of bleeding esophageal varices.

Occasionally, small venous connections open up between the splenic hilum and left renal vein, with resulting portosystemic drainage directly into the inferior vena cava (spontaneous splenorenal shunt). Less frequently, the umbilical vein, which passes through the falciform ligament and ligamentum teres from the porta hepatis to the umbilical vein, recanalizes (Cruveilhier-Baumgarten syndrome). In its advanced stage, this collateral circulation (Fig. 31.2) can produce dilated and markedly tortuous subcutaneous periumbilical veins referred to as "caput medusae." In questionable cases, color duplex sonography can be used to detect a decreased or reversed (hepatofugal) portal blood flow.

The evaluation of the porta hepatis should not only assess the luminal diameter of the portal vein, but should also exclude enlarged periportal lymph nodes (55) (Fig. 31.3) by systematically scrutinizing the periportal region. Inflammatory nodal enlargement frequently accompanies viral hepatitis, cholecystitis or pancreatitis and, if present, should lead to the evaluation of other nodal areas and spleen size to be used as baseline for follow-up examinations to determine progression or regression of the disease process.

Checklist for portal hypertension:

- Detection of portocaval collaterals at the porta hepatis
- Diameter of the portal vein ≥ 15 mm
- Dilation of the splenic vein > 12 mm
- Splenomegaly
- Detection of ascites
- Recanalized umbilical vein (Cruveilhier-Baumgarten syndrome)
- Esophageal varices (bleeding)

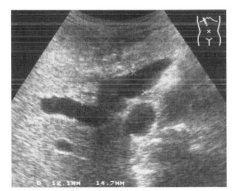

Fig. 31.1 a

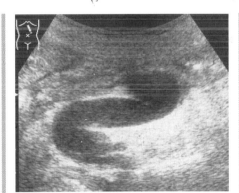

Fig. 31.2 a

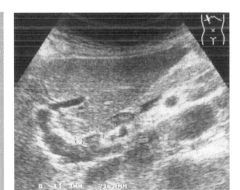

Fig. 31.3 a

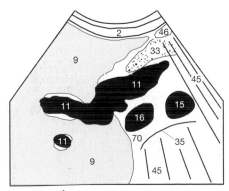

Fig. 31.1 b

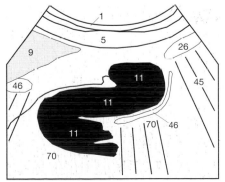

Fig. 31.2 b

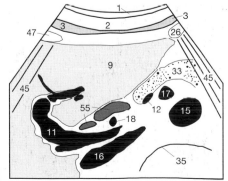

Fig. 31.3 b

After this session, the easily comprehensible sagittal and transverse sections are supplemented by oblique sections, rendering the spatial orientation of individual structures that is much more demanding. It is in your best interest not to begin with Lesson 3 until you have mastered the answers to the following questions – even if some effort is involved.

Here is a tip for time management: Do not spend more than two minutes for each exercise (you will not retain anything thereafter anyhow). Allow at least two hours between the exercises and do other things in between (interval method). Correct your answers critically and do not give up too easily.

1. Take a separate sheet of paper and, entirely from memory (without consulting this workbook or any other material), draw the approximate course of the relevant upper abdominal vessels in relation to each other and to the pancreas. Annotate each structure with the customary abbreviations. Compare your drawing with **Figures 25.2** and **25.3**. Resolve any uncertainty or deficiency by comparing your work to the legends found on the back cover flap. Repeat this exercise in the spirit of self-improvement until you succeed without making any mistakes.

2. Enhance and anchor your knowledge of the sectional anatomy by drawing (from memory, of course) the standard transverse sections through the celiac axis and through the crossing renal veins. Compare your sketches with the drawings shown on page 110. **Long term**, you only will remember structures you can correctly outline in position and size.

Level of the celiac axis   Level of the crossing renal vein

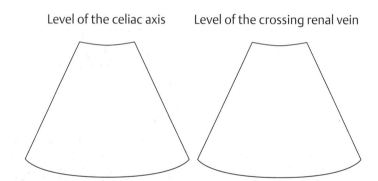

3. How does the echogenicity of the pancreatic parenchyma increase with advancing age and obesity? What trick do you know to improve the delineation of the tail of the pancreas? What other image modalities are available to investigate the pancreas?

4. On the image shown in **Figure 32.1**, name every vessel and every other structure. Which vessel appears dilated or congested? What can be the cause? Is this finding pathologic?

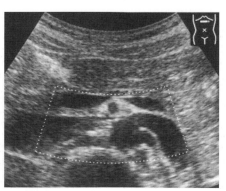

Fig. 32.1

Q

Lesson 3 deals with the liver and gallbladder. Both organs should be thoroughly (!) scanned in two planes in deep inspiration. We recommend always following a standard pattern, beginning with a sagittal section that uses the inferior vena cava (IVC) as a demarcation line, as shown in **Fig. 19.3**. From there, the left hepatic lobe is scanned laterally back and forth. After expiration and another deep breath, the right hepatic lobe is scanned the same way with slow and continuous tilting of the probe **(Fig. 33.1.a)**. The visualization of the cranial, subdiaphragmatic sections of the liver is a major challenge, which can be met by asking the patient to take a really deep breath and by adequate tilting of the probe **(Fig. 33.1b)**. Because of the large size of the right lobe, this maneuver generally must be used once for the cranial sections and – after the patient catches his/her breath – again for the inferior sections. Do not forget to reduce the magnification to have the posterior hepatic sections included in the image. Keep in mind that the portovenous branches **(11)** in the hepatic parenchyma **(9)** are always surrounded by a hyperechoic rim related to accompanying biliary ducts, arteries and periportal connective tissue. In contrast, the hepatic veins **(10)** are usually visualized without a hyperechoic border.

The determination of liver size has become less important in recent years because of its poor reliability. Typically, the craniocaudal and anteroposterior diameters were measured in the sagittal plane along the right MCL **(Fig. 33.2)**. The normal craniocaudal diameter measures between 11 and 15 cm in adults, but varies strongly with the depth of inspiration because of the elastic adaptation of the hepatic parenchyma to the thoracic cavity **(9)**. More reliable is the assessment of the inferior marginal angle of the right hepatic lobe, which should be less than 45 degrees. The inferior hepatic margin appears rounded if the liver is congested or enlarged for any other reason. The lateral marginal angle of the left lobe should be less than 30 degrees and normally is more acute than the caudal hepatic margin.

The gallbladder **(14)** can be evaluated together with the inferior hepatic margin. The evaluation of the gallbladder should be done preprandially **(Fig. 33.3)**, since this allows a better assessment of its wall thickness **(80)**, which should not exceed 4 mm preprandially. Postprandially, the contracted gallbladder precludes the exclusion of edematous wall thickening, stones, polyps or tumors (see pages 43, 44).

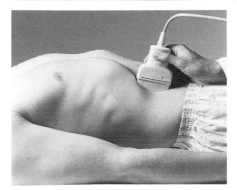

Fig. 33.1 a

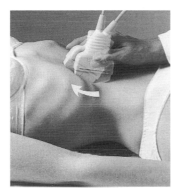

Fig. 33.1 b

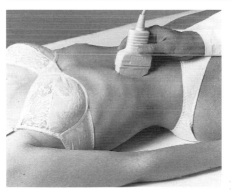

Fig. 33.2 a

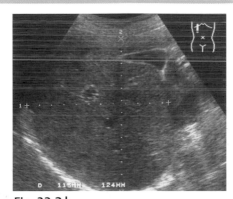

Fig. 33.2 b

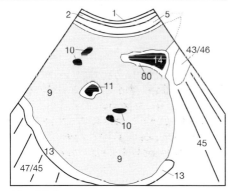

Fig. 33.2 c

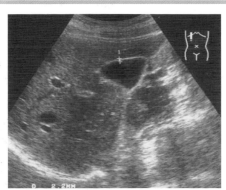

Fig. 33.3 a

Fig. 33.3 b

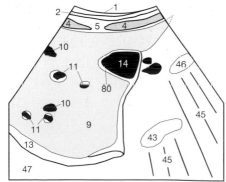

Fig. 33.3 c

After sagittal scanning of the liver, the left hepatic lobe too is systematically scanned craniocaudally in the transverse plane. It is most practical to examine the right hepatic lobe in subcostal oblique sections parallel to the right costal arch (**Fig. 34.1**). What mistake is most commonly made here when holding the probe? The answer is in the lower left-hand corner of this page.

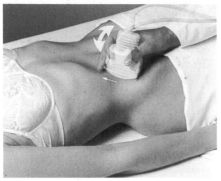

Fig. 34.1

Hepatic Venous Star

The plane of the right subcostal oblique section (**Fig. 34.2a**) is especially suitable for the lengthwise visualization of the hepatic veins (**10**) to their confluence with the obliquely sectioned and therefore oval-shaped inferior vena cava (**16**). This elongated, straight course of the hepatic veins is typical and only altered by focal intrahepatic lesions or right heart failure.

Right Heart Failure

In case of a borderline diameter of the inferior vena cava and inconclusive testing for caval collapse with forced inspiration, the diameter of the peripheral hepatic veins can be used as an additional criterion for right heart failure. The maximal diameter of a peripheral hepatic vein (seen in the left upper region of the image) should not exceed 6 mm. Measuring the hepatic veins at the confluence with the vena cava (**16**) has the disadvantage of wide anatomic variations. Up to 10 to 12 mm can still be entirely normal. **Figure 34.3** shows the typical manifestation of an overt right heart failure with congested and bulging hepatic veins and bulging inferior vena cava (**16**).

Please note that the right hepatic vein runs perpendicular to the direction of the sound waves in this plane and can show a thin hyperechoic wall that is otherwise only seen in portal vein branches (**11**) (**Fig. 34.2b**). Furthermore, this plane is very well suited to evaluate the hepatic veins for a clinically suspected thrombosis with duplex color sonography. In any case, check the peripheral hepatic sections for possible rarefied vascularity as an indirect sign of a cirrhotic transformation of the hepatic parenchyma.

This image plane can also confirm a right pleural effusion behind (on the image below) the hyperechoic diaphragm (**13**), where normally only acoustic shadows (**45**) behind pulmonary air (**47**) or a mirror artifact of the hepatic parenchyma (**9**) is identified.

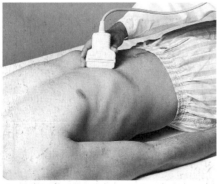

Fig. 34.2 a

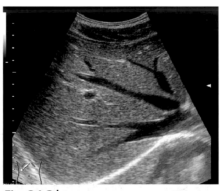

Fig. 34.2 b

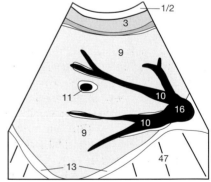

Fig. 34.2 c

Normal Values:
Hepatic veins: < 6 mm
(periphery)

Answer to Fig. 34.1:
The transducer is positioned too far lateroinferiorly. It must be moved medially and closer to the costal arch (see small arrow).

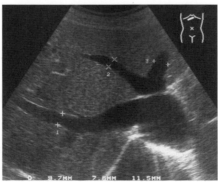

Fig. 34.3 a

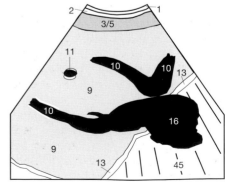

Fig. 34.3 b

Systemic scrutiny of the liver can bring out normal variants that mimic focal lesions. In physically well-trained patients, for instance, hyperechoic structures (↓) that appear to arise from the concave diaphragmatic surface (13) can indent the hepatic dome (9) (Fig. 35.1). These pseudo-lesions represent thickened muscular bands that produce cord-like imprints on the liver while extending from the central tendon to the costal and lumbar insertion of the diaphragm.

They have no clinical significance and should not be mistaken for patho-logic processes. A diaphragmatic mus-cular band (13) can also be singular (Fig. 35.2) and project as a mirror artifact (51) along the pulmonary side (47) of the diaphragm (see page 15).

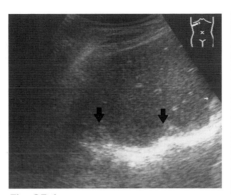

Fig. 35.1 a

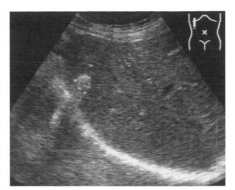

Fig. 35.2 a

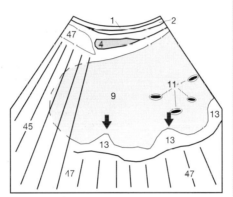

Fig. 35.1 b

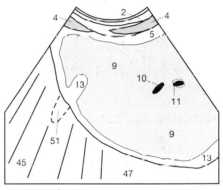

Fig. 35.2 b

Fatty Liver

A fatty liver or hepatic steatosis produces a diffusely increased echogenicity of the liver (Fig. 35.3). This increase in echogenicity is best appreciated when compared with the echogenicity of the adjacent kidney (29). In normal patients, liver and kidney exhibit about the same echogenicity (Fig. 45.3). In severe hepatic fatty infiltration, the parenchymal sound reflection can be so pronounced (9) that the liver can barely be evaluated with increasing distance from the transducer. Though sound enhancement (70) is evident behind the gallbladder (14) (Fig. 35.4), the posterior hepatic regions along the lower border of the image are no longer discernible despite depth gain compensation.

Do you remember the reason underlying the phenomenon of posterior sound enhancement? If not, look it up again on page 14.

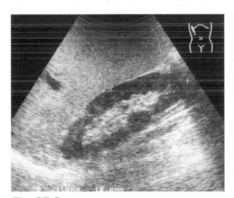

Fig. 35.3 a

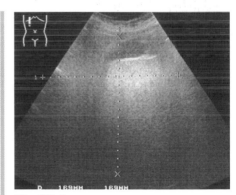

Fig. 35.4 a

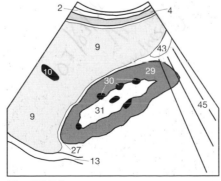

Fig. 35.3 b

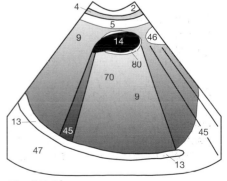

Fig. 35.4 b

Focally Increased Deposition of Fat

Fatty infiltration does not necessarily occur throughout the entire liver; it can be confined to selected hepatic areas. Sites predisposed to focal fatty changes (63) are around the gallbladder fossa or anterior to the portal vein (11). The areas of increased fat content are sharply demarcated and more echogenic than the surrounding hepatic parenchyma (9). They can assume bizarre geographic configurations (Fig. 36.1) but lack any space-occupying effect. Adjacent hepatic veins (10) or the branches of the portal veins (11) are **not** displaced.

These areas of focal fatty infiltration must be distinguished from the falciform ligament (8). Its connective tissue and surrounding fat can produce a similar hyperechoic structure that sharply interrupts the adjacent normal hepatic parenchyma (Fig. 36.2).

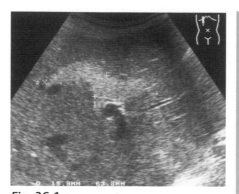

Fig. 36.1 a

Fig. 36.2 a

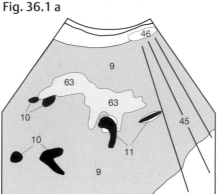

Fig. 36.1 b

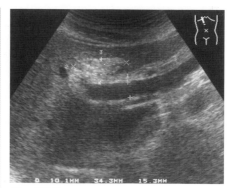

Fig. 36.2 b

Focally Decreased Deposition of Fat

Fatty infiltration might also spare certain hepatic areas, creating focal areas of less deposited fat (62). These regions of reduced fat content are primarily found in the immediate vicinity of the portal vein or gallbladder (14) (Fig. 36.4). It is important to keep in mind that this finding again lacks a space-occupying component. Adjacent hepatic veins (10) are not displaced (Fig. 36.3) and stay their course. Peripherally located areas of spared fatty infiltration show no bulging hepatic border and do not project into the gallbladder, as frequently seen with tumors or metastases. The branches of the portal vein (11) can be distinguished from hepatic veins by their hyperechoic outline. This so-called "reinforced river embankment" is caused by impedance jumps between the walls of the portal vein branches and the accompanying biliary ducts and hepatic arteries. The accentuated hyperechogenicity of the portal vein wall (5) in the vicinity of the porta hepatis (Fig. 36.2) should not be mistaken for focal fatty infiltration. Since the hepatic veins (10) traverse the parenchyma without concomitant vessels, they lack this impedance jump. Only large hepatic veins perpendicular to the sound beam can be accompanied by a hyperechoic wall (see page 34).

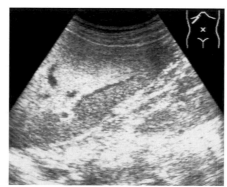

Fig. 36.3 a

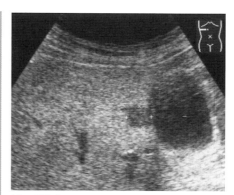

Fig. 36.4 a

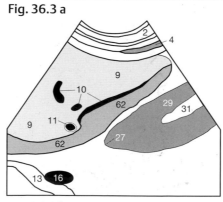

Fig. 36.3 b

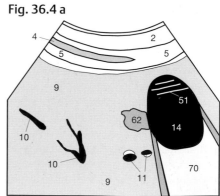

Fig. 36.4 b

The most frequent focal lesions of the liver are benign cysts **(64)**. These can be congenital (dysontogenetic) or acquired. In contrast to congenital biliary dilation (Caroli syndrome), congenital cysts contain no bile, but serous fluid **(Fig. 37.1)**. Since they are filled with homogeneous fluid, they are anechoic unless they have bled. They generally are clinically irrelevant.

Cyst Criteria

The criteria differentiating benign cysts from other hypoechoic lesions include anechoic content, spherical shape, sharp demarcation, smooth outline and, with larger cysts, distal acoustic enhancement (see page 14), as well as a possible edge effect (see page 15) and accentuated entrance and exit echoes (where the sound waves hit the cysts at a 90-degree angle). Diagnostic difficulties can arise when internal echoes are found secondary to intracystic hemorrhage. Furthermore, these hemorrhagic cysts can exhibit indentations or delicate septa. Parasitic hepatic cysts must then be excluded **(Fig. 37.4)**.

The most frequent parasitic involvement of the liver is cystic echinococcal disease (Echinococcus cysticus), which characteristically produces several daughter cysts within a large cyst. Such hydatid cysts should not be aspirated to avoid possible rupture with subsequent seeding of the larvae. The identification of the less frequent alveolar echinococcal disease (Echinococcus alveolaris) is sonographically more difficult. A mixed solid, liquid and cystic space-occupying lesion is typically found **(54) (Fig. 37.4a)**. Its differentiation from primary hepatocellular carcinoma, metastasis **(Fig.40.3)**, abscess or old hematoma is virtually impossible.

Hepatic Hemangiomas (61) are homogeneously hyperechoic (bright) in comparison to the adjacent hepatic tissue **(9)**, have a smooth outline, and lack a hypoechoic rim **(Fig. 37.2)**. A draining but not dilated hepatic vein **(10)** can be characteristically found in the immediate vicinity **(Fig. 37.3)**. Most hepatic hemangiomas are small **(Fig. 37.2)** but can be multifocal and quite large. The larger hemangiomas often become heterogeneous, making it difficult to differentiate them from other tumors and requiring CT for further evaluation.

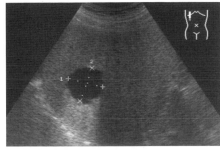

Fig. 37.1 a

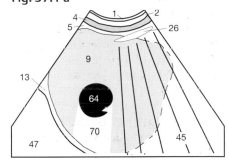

Fig. 37.1 b

Checklist of cyst criteria

- Spherical shape
- Anechoic content
- Sharp demarcation
- Posterior acoustic enhancement
- Edge effect
- Accentuated entrance / exit echo

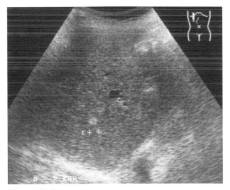

Fig. 37.2 a

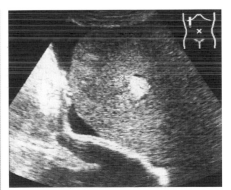

Fig. 37.3 a

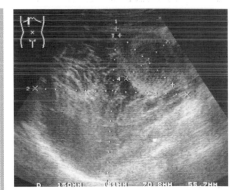

Fig. 37.4 a

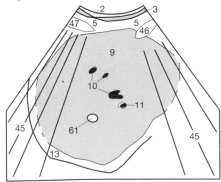

Fig. 37.2 b

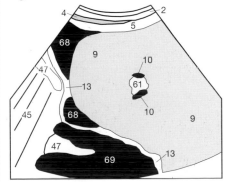

Fig. 37.3 b

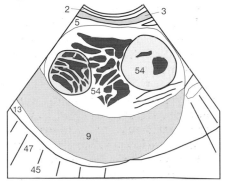

Fig. 37.4 b

Inflammatory hepatic processes include cholangitis, fungal disease in immunosuppressed patients or hematogenous seeding. The sonographic findings exhibit quite a variable morphology.

Depending on stage and immune state, hepatic abscesses **(58)** can have an anechoic center due to liquefaction **(Fig. 38.2)** or heterogeneous areas surrounded by a hypoechoic rim, or even present as hyperechoic lesions **(Fig. 38.1)**. The variable appearance of abscesses makes their differentiation from heterogeneous focal nodular hyperplasia (FNH) **(Fig. 38.3)** or malignant tumors difficult. FNH is a primary benign hepatic tumor that has a predilection for women using oral birth contraception. Special examination techniques with contrast media can bring out a typical stellate figure in its center during the early angiographic phase **(Fig. 38.4)**. Spiral CT can differentiate inconclusive cases from large hetero-geneous hemangiomas: Following bolus injection of contrast media, hemangiomas show a so-called "iris aperture phenomenon." The contrast enhancement progresses centripetally from the outside to the inside, producing a target-like pattern (target sign) **(Fig. 38.5)**.

Hepatic tumors can have an intrahepatic space-occupying effect and compress adjacent hepatic tissue. If the compression of adjacent biliary ducts has led to obstruction (cholestasis), bile can be temporarily drained by internal stents into the duodenum or through percutaneous transhepatic catheters into a collection bag. The effectiveness of inserted drainage catheters **(59)** can be easily monitored by follow-up sonographic examinations **(Fig. 38.1)**.

Pneumobilia

Occasionally, air bubbles **(60)** can be observed in the biliary ducts **(66)**, caused by infection or preceding ERCP as well as by previous papillotomy or biliary-enteric anastomosis **(Fig. 38.2)**. The acronym **ERCP** stands for **e**ndoscopic **r**etrograde **c**holangio**p**ancreatography. Through a gastroscope advanced into the duodenum to the major papilla (papilla of Vater), a second "baby endoscope" is inserted into the distal common bile duct. A papillotomy is an incision through a scarred papilla.

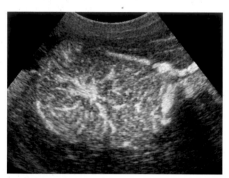

Fig. 38.4 (Dietrich, M.D., Frankfurt)

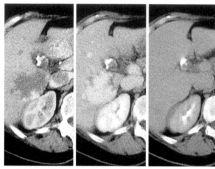

Fig. 38.5

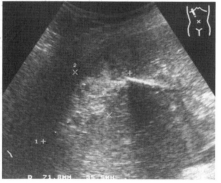

Fig. 38.1 a

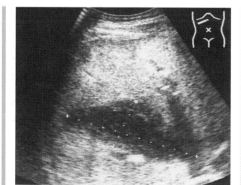

Fig. 38.2 a

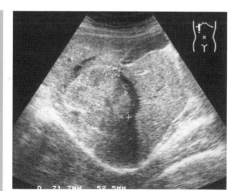

Fig. 38.3 a

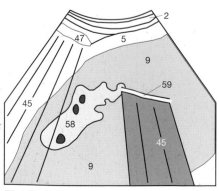

Fig. 38.1 b

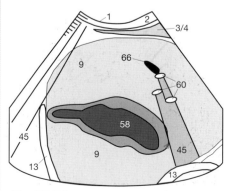

Fig. 38.2 b

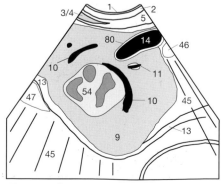

Fig. 38.3 b

In addition to chronic alcoholism, possible causes of cirrhosis include viral hepatitis, metabolic disorders and exposure to toxic substances in the environment. Latent cirrhosis without hepatic decompensation can lack sonographically detectable changes and, consequently, cirrhosis cannot definitively be excluded by sonography alone. However, several criteria exist for more advanced stages of cirrhosis.

Cirrhosis Criteria

While the normal liver (9) exhibits a thin echogenic capsule along its border (**Fig. 33.3**), the cirrhotic liver has an irregular surface with small undulations or bumps. This causes increased scattering of the sound beam, and only few sound waves reflected from the capsule return to the transducer. This results in only patchy or no visualization of the capsule. The absence of a capsular line is best appreciated with ascites (68) around the liver (**Fig. 39.1**). Furthermore, cirrhosis rarefies the peripheral vasculature (**Fig. 39.1**), with the remaining visualized vessels showing variable diameters and wider confluence angles (> 45°). Normal hepatic veins (10) follow a straight course, join each other at an acute angle and are traceable to the hepatic periphery (**Fig. 34.2**).

In cirrhosis, the branches of the portal vein close to the porta hepatis often show more prominent hyperechoic walls, i.e., a more apparent "reinforced embankment," and sudden caliber changes referred to as "pruned portal tree." Regenerating nodules exhibit normal echogenicity and can only be indirectly recognized by displaced adjacent vessels. Other findings suggestive of cirrhosis are deformed and biconvex hepatic configuration, decreased pliability when pressing the transducer over the liver, and an enlarged and rounded left or caudate lobe.

Complications of Cirrhosis

Possible sequelae of cirrhosis include portal hypertension (see page 31), ascites (68) and hepatocellular carcinomas (54) on the basis of a long-standing cirrhosis (**Fig. 39.2**). Therefore, a cirrhotic liver must be carefully and thoroughly (!) scrutinized for focal space-occupying lesions. Only the late cirrhotic stage produces a shrunken liver (**Fig. 39.2**). Hepatocellular carcinomas (54) can be isoechoic with the remaining hepatic parenchyma (9) and might only be indirectly detectable by secondary convex displacement of neighboring hepatic veins (10) (**Fig. 39.3**).

Checklist of cirrhosis criteria
- Absence of the thin echogenic capsular line
- Peripheral vascular rarefaction
- Widened angle of the hepatic veins > 45 degrees
- Sudden caliber changes of the portal vein
- Possibly more conspicuous "reinforced embankment" of the portal vein
- Regenerating nodules with displaced vessels

Additional findings in the late stage
- Rounded organ shape (obtuse marginal angles)
- Shrunken liver
- Signs of portal hypertension

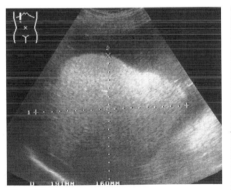

Fig. 39.1 a

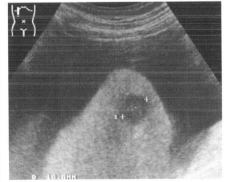

Fig. 39.2 a

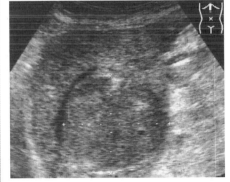

Fig. 39.3 a

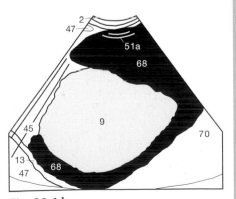

Fig. 39.1 b

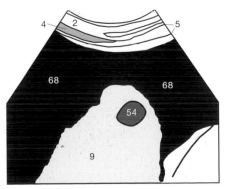

Fig. 39.2 b

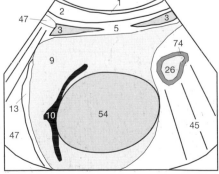

Fig. 39.3 b

Secondary neoplastic lesions (metastases) in the liver do not only arise from primary tumors of the gastrointestinal tract, but also from primary tumors of the breast and lung. The sonographic findings are polymorphic. Hepatic metastases (56) from colorectal carcinomas are often hyperechoic (Fig. 40.2), presumably related to neovascularity secondary to their relatively slow growth. The more rapidly growing metastases from bronchogenic or mammary carcinomas consist almost exclusively of tumor cells that have the tendency to be more hypoechoic. In view of their multifarious presentation, metastases cannot be reliably assigned to any particular primary tumor, even though color duplex sonography with visualization of the vascular architecture and elasticity imaging recently have shown a promising approach to the differential diagnostic evaluation.

Characteristically, metastases (56) exhibit a hypoechoic halo or rim, as seen in Figures 40.1 and 40.2. This hypoechoic halo could represent either an active proliferating tumor zone or perifocal edema. Central necrosis (57) can be seen as cystic areas caused by liquefaction due to rapid tumor growth or chemotherapy (Fig. 40.3).

Large metastases are generally marked by their space-occupying effect, with displaced adjacent vessels and compressed biliary ducts that can lead to regional intrahepatic cholestasis (Fig. 41.2). Peripherally located metastases can focally expand the hepatic contour, easily seen with laparoscopy.

Chemotherapy can induce variable signs of tumor regression depending on the therapeutic effect. These include heterogeneous scars, calcifications or partial cystic liquefaction. Such regressively altered metastases or small metastatic nodules cannot be easily separated from areas of cirrhotic transformation. It is crucial to follow these findings sonographically to assess their growth potential. Alternatively, percutaneous needle biopsy can be obtained under ultrasound or CT guidance. Multiple metastases of different sizes and echogenicities suggest hematogenous spreading at different times.

Quiz – Test Yourself:

Use the images on this page to test your basic knowledge. Do you remember why hypoechoic (dark) bands (45) traverse the liver in Figure 40.1 and why the region between both bands (70) is somewhat more hyperechoic (brighter) than the remaining hepatic parenchyma (9)? Just keep in mind that the gallbladder (14) is located between both artifacts and the transducer and that the sound beam hits the gallbladder wall (80) tangentially. If you still cannot come up with a satisfactory explanation, you should go back to pages 14 and 15 and study the material found there once more.

On the subject of images: In Figure 37.3a, three pages back, didn't you notice anechoic (black) areas that defy a physiologic explanation? Unless you have already come up with an explanation, please have another look at the image. A solution to this puzzle can be found on page 109.

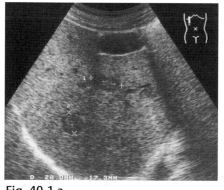

Fig. 40.1 a

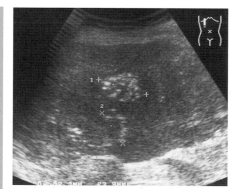

Fig. 40.2 a

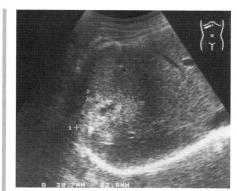

Fig. 40.3 a

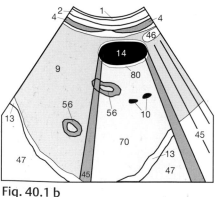

Fig. 40.1 b

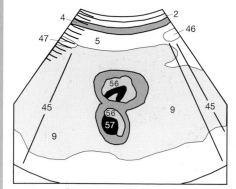

Fig. 40.2 b

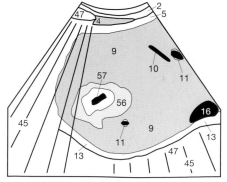

Fig. 40.3 b

At the level of the minor omentum, the common bile duct **(66)** normally measures up to 6 mm, but luminal diameters between 7 and 9 mm are still within the normal range **(Fig. 41.1)**, particularly after cholecystectomy. A dilated duct (exceeding 9 mm in diameter) invariably becomes visible anterolaterally to (in the image above) the portal vein **(11)** (see page 30). Even when the distal segment of the common bile duct is obscured by duodenal air **(Fig. 25.3)**, a proximal obstruction (e.g., hepatic metastases with intrahepatic biliary duct obstruction) can be sonographically distinguished from distal obstruction (e.g., a gallstone lodged at the papilla or a carcinoma of the head of the pancreas). A proximal obstruction distends neither the gallbladder **(14)** nor the common bile duct.

Obstructive Cholestasis

The small intrahepatic biliary ducts run parallel to the portal vein branches **(11)** and are normally tiny or even invisible. The ductal dilation caused by biliary obstruction brings out these small ducts along the portal veins, creating the "double-barrel shotgun sign" **(Figs. 41.2 and 42.3)**. In up to 90% of such cases, sonography succeeds in distinguishing between obstructive (ductal dilation) and hepatocellular (without ductal dilation) cholestasis.

Severe mechanical biliary obstruction **(Fig. 41.2)** characteristically produces a tortuous dilation of the intrahepatic biliary ducts **(66)** resembling a "towering antler." The cholestasis-induced increased viscosity can lead to crystalline precipitation of the bile **(Fig. 41.3)**. This so-called "sludge" **(67)** can also be seen after prolonged fasting without biliary obstruction.

Before making the diagnosis of sludge, a thickness artifact (see page 14) should be excluded by obtaining additional sections and by moving and turning the patient. For persistent inconclusive findings, one might try to disperse the presumed sludge with the transducer. A biliary obstruction can be drained by inserting a biliary stent **(59)** as part of an **ERCP** (endoscopic retrograde cholangiopancreatography). Alternatively, biliary drainage can be achieved by placing a percutaneous transhepatic catheter.

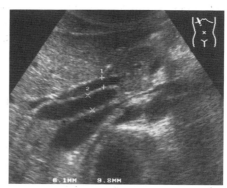

Fig. 41.1 a

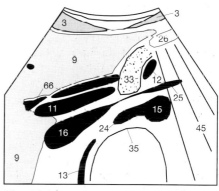

Fig. 41.1 b

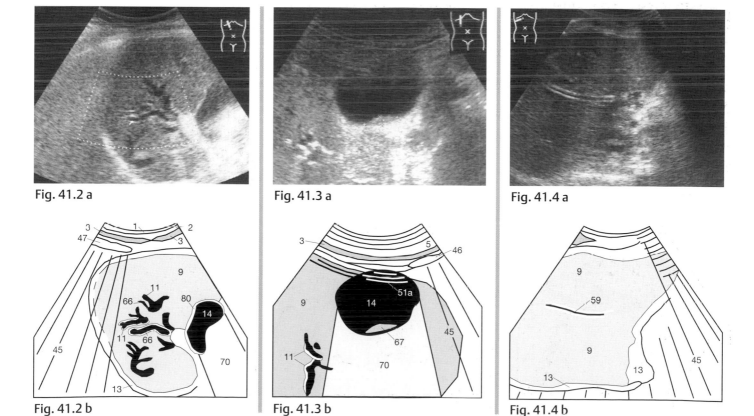

Fig. 41.2 a

Fig. 41.3 a

Fig. 41.4 a

Fig. 41.2 b

Fig. 41.3 b

Fig. 41.4 b

Stones in the gallbladder (gallstones) form because of a shift in the composition of the excreted bile. Depending on their components, gallstones **(49)** can have almost total sound transmission and be visible **(Fig. 42.3)**, float within the gallbladder (cholesterol stones), or have such a strong calciuminduced sound reflection that only the surface near the transducer can be visualized **(Fig. 42.1)**.

A stone is easily diagnosed and clearly differentiated from a polyp **(65)** as long as it can be dislodged from the gallbladder wall **(80)** by moving and turning the patient **(Fig. 42.2)**. Some stones, however, can remain fixed on the gallbladder wall due to previous inflammatory processes or become lodged in the infundibulum, rendering the differentiation between stones and polyps difficult.

Acoustic shadowing **(45)** distal to such a lesion **(Figs. 42.1** and **42.3)** also favors a stone. An edge effect of the gallbladder wall **(45** in **Fig. 42.2)** must be carefully distinguished from a stone-induced acoustic shadow (see page 15) to avoid any misinterpretation. **Figure 42.2** shows mural polyps without acoustic shadowing but with adjacent edge effects. Such polyps should be followed for growth to detect any malignant process early or to remove them preemptively before malignant transformation.

Intrahepatic cholestasis **(Fig. 41.2)** is not necessarily a manifestation of malignancy. It can also be caused by obstructing gallstones **(49)** in the intrahepatic ducts **(66)** **(Fig. 42.3)**.

The prevalence of cholelithiasis is about 15%, with older women more often affected. Since 80% of patients with gallstones are asymptomatic, only the complications of detected gallstones are consequential (cholecystitis, cholangitis, colic, biliary obstruction). Stone removal can be achieved by percutaneous or open cholecystectomy or, alternatively, by **ESWL** (**e**xtracorporeal **s**hock **w**ave **l**ithotripsy) or ERCP (see page 38). Furthermore, the composition of the bile can be altered by medication, and some stones regress following dietary changes.

Note the thin, single-layered, echogenic wall **(80)** of both gallbladders **(14)** shown in **Figures 42.1** and **42.2**. Inflammatory thickening of the gallbladder wall is absent. To make wall thickening and intraluminal processes detectable, the sonographic examination of the gallbladder should be obtained with the patient NPO. Postprandial contraction of the gallbladder precludes an adequate evaluation of its lumen. Images of typical cases of an inflamed gallbladder (cholecystitis) are shown on the next page.

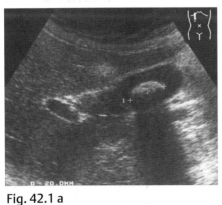

Fig. 42.1 a

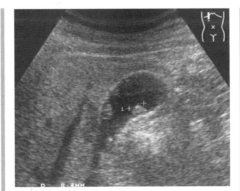

Fig. 42.2 a

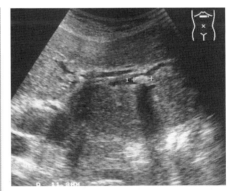

Fig. 42.3 a

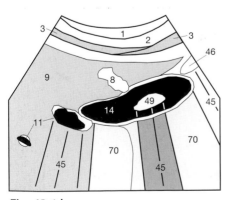

Fig. 42.1 b

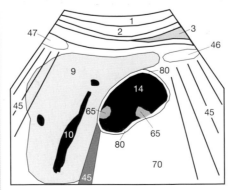

Fig. 42.2 b

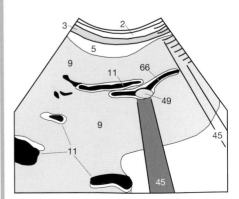

Fig. 42.3 b

The normal gallbladder (14) has a thin, single-layered wall (80), measuring less than 4 mm preprandially (Fig. 43.3). Cholecystitis is invariably caused by stones (49) in the gallbladder. A tender gallbladder can be the only finding in early cholecystitis, but this is soon followed by inflammatory mural edema with thickening and a multilayered appearance of the gallbladder wall (80) (Fig. 43.1).

Gallbladder wall thickening can be seen in ascites (68) without inflammatory wall thickening. This can also be caused by right heart failure or hypoalbuminemia (Fig. 43.2).

An additional finding indicative of an acute inflammation is pericholecystic accumulation of fluid (68). In some cases, the accumulated fluid can be confined to Morison's pouch between the inferior hepatic border and the right kidney. Finally, the gallbladder outline can become indistinct along the hepatic parenchyma (9). A transverse diameter of the gallbladder of more than 4 cm indicates a hydrops, but even more characteristic is the change from a typical pear shape to an apple shape due to biconvex and spherical expansion of the gallbladder.

It is crucial to recognize any air within the lumen of the gallbladder or in its wall (mural emphysema), since an infection with gas-forming organisms implies a bad prognosis and is associated with a high risk of perforation. Chronic cholecystitis can lead to a contracted gallbladder or porcelain gallbladder. Both conditions are often difficult to differentiate by sonography. A completely calcified gallbladder wall can reflect sound waves like air in the hepatic colon flexure, explaining why a porcelain gallbladder is easily missed sonographically. Clinical findings or supplemental CT often provide further guidance in these cases.

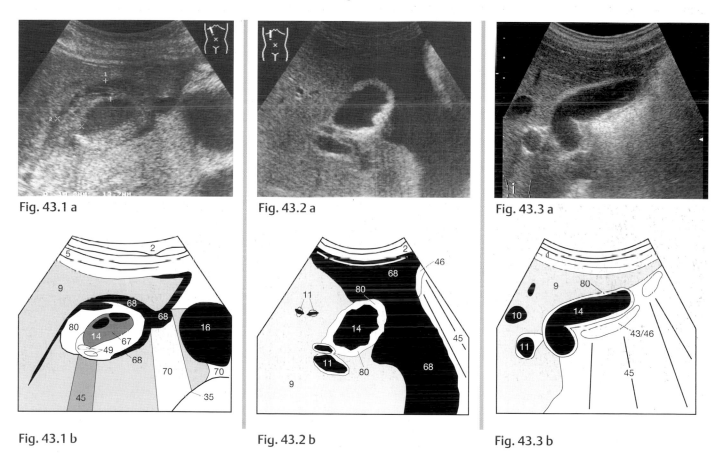

Fig. 43.1 a   Fig. 43.2 a   Fig. 43.3 a

Fig. 43.1 b   Fig. 43.2 b   Fig. 43.3 b

Please take this quiz to test how familiar you are with the material presented in Lesson 3. You will find the answers to the questions on the preceding pages and the answers to the image quiz on page 107. Check the answers only after you have worked on all questions – getting the answers too early ruins the suspense and defeats the purpose of this quiz.

1. Repeat the drawing of the standard image plane of the porta hepatis. Where are hepatic artery and bile duct in relation to the portal vein and inferior vena cava? Compare your drawing with **Figure 30.2c**.

2. What is the name of the sonographic section that visualizes the hepatic venous star? How do you hold the transducer to obtain this plane? Draw the corresponding body markers and draw the appearance of the hepatic venous star. What can be measured at what level? Why?

3. Write down the six characteristic findings of portal hypertension and the eight characteristic findings of cirrhosis. Compare your answers with the checklists on pages 31 and 39, and repeat this exercise for several days until you do not overlook any finding (leave time to rest in between!).

4. Do you remember the preferred sites for focally decreased and focally increased fatty infiltration of the liver? How can they be differentiated from malignant hepatic processes?

5. Review the following four sonographic images. Write down the image planes, visualized organs and vessels, and your differential diagnosis. Include **all** abnormalities, since some images display **several** pathologic processes.

6. What is the maximum diameter of the common bile duct? What diameter in mm is suspicious for a biliary obstruction?

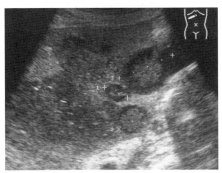

Fig. 44.1

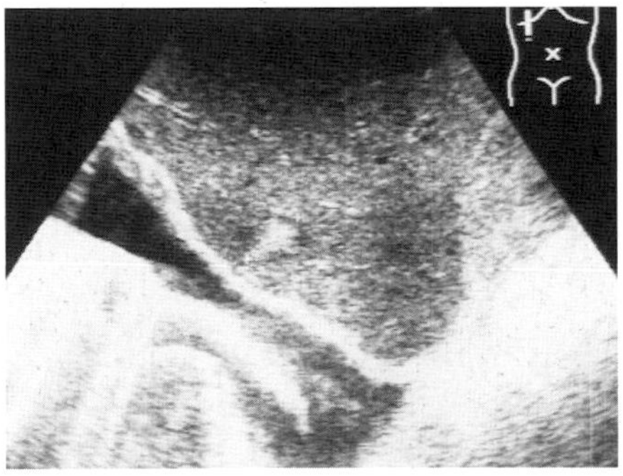

Fig. 44.2

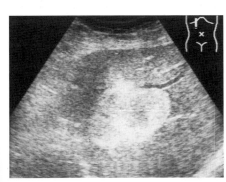

Fig. 44.3

7. Write down several differential diagnoses for **Figure 44.4**. The solution is on page 107.

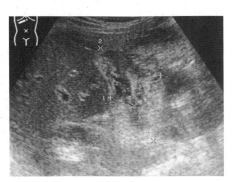

Fig. 44.4

Q

The right kidney can often be well visualized longitudinally through the liver from the anterior axillary line, with the patient supine and taking a deep breath (**Fig. 45.2a**). Alternatively, the transducer can be placed parallel to the intercostal spaces with the patient in the left lateral decubitus position (**Fig. 45.1a**). Each kidney should be scanned systematically in two planes. The left kidney can be visualized in transverse and longitudinal sections with the patient supine or in the right lateral decubitus position. With deep inspiration, the kidney moves craniocaudally along the psoas (**44**) by 3 to 7 cm. This displacement can be used to position the kidneys in a better acoustic window, avoiding interfering ribs and intestinal air.

Normally, the parenchyma of the right kidney is isoechoic with the hepatic parenchyma (**Fig. 45.3**). It should measure at least 1.3 cm in width. The typical longitudinal section (**Fig. 45.2**) displays the hypoechoic medullary pyramids (**30**) like a string of pearls between the parenchymal cortex (**29**) and the central hyperechoic collecting system. They should not be mistaken for anechoic cysts or calices. The echogenicity of the central renal components is caused by impedance jumps between vascular walls, linings of the collecting system, fatty tissue and connective tissue.

The transverse section (**Fig. 45.3**) delineates the right renal hilum, together with the renal vein (**25**) as it extends to the inferior vena cava (**16**). The hyperechoic suprarenal fat capsule around the upper renal pole (**27**) must be scrutinized for a hypoechoic space-occupying lesion, which might represent an adrenal tumor. An important measurement for chronic renal diseases is the ratio between the width of the peripheral hypoechoic parenchyma and the width of the central hyperechoic pelvic complex. This so-called parenchyma-pelvis index (PPI) increases with age (see Table):

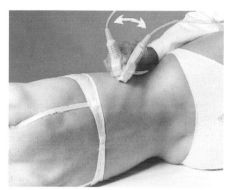

Fig. 45.1 a

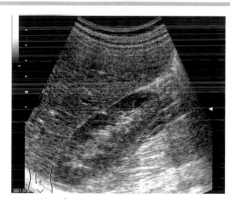

Fig. 45.1 b

Checklist of Normal Renal Values:

Renal length:	10 – 12 cm
Renal width:	4 – 6 cm
Respiratory mobility:	3 – 7 cm
Parenchymal width:	1.3 – 2.5 cm

PP-Index	age < 30 years	> 1.6 : 1
PP-Index	age 30-60 years	1.2–1.6 : 1
PP-Index	age > 60 years	1.1 : 1

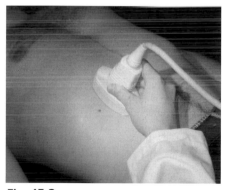

Fig. 45.2 a

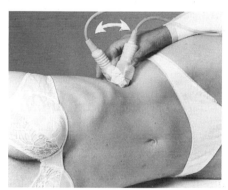

Fig. 45.2 b

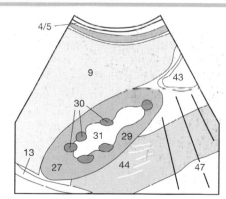

Fig. 45.2 c

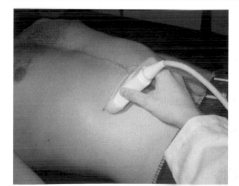

Fig. 45.3 a

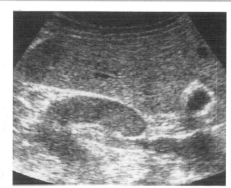

Fig. 45.3 b

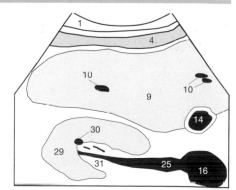

Fig. 45.3 c

Normal Variants

The normal configuration of the kidney (**Fig. 45.2**) can show several changes related to its embryologic development. Hyperplastic columns of Bertini, which do not differ in echogenicity from the remaining renal parenchyma, can protrude from the parenchyma (**29**) into the renal pelvis (**31**). An isoechoic parenchymal bridge can completely divide the collecting system. A partial or complete parenchymal gap at the same location indicates a renal duplication (**Fig. 46.1**) with separate ureters and blood supply for each moiety.

The prevertebral parenchymal bridge of horseshoe kidneys might be, at first glance, mistaken for preaortic lymphadenopathy or a thrombosed aortic aneurysm. A lobulated renal contour can be seen in children and young adults as manifestation of persistent fetal lobulation, characterized by an otherwise smooth renal surface indented between the individual medullary pyramids. These changes must be differentiated from the more triangular scars after renal infarcts (**Fig. 54.3**), which can be found mainly in older patients with atherosclerotic stenosis of the renal artery or suprarenal aortic aneurysm.

About 10% of patients show a localized parenchymal thickening along the lateral border of the left kidney, usually just below the inferior pole of the spleen. This is an anatomic variant and generally referred to as "dromedary hump." Occasionally, its differentiation from a true renal tumor can be difficult.

Renal Cysts

Like hepatic cysts (see page 37), dysontogenetic renal cysts (**64**) generally are anechoic and, when exceeding a certain size, produce distal acoustic enhancement (**70**), as shown in **Figure 46.2**. Do you remember the other cyst criteria allowing the differentiation from hypoechoic renal tumors in obese patients? If not, you know where to find the answer.

Cysts can be separated into peripheral cysts projecting from the renal surface, parenchymal cysts (**Fig. 46.2**), and peripelvic cysts, with the latter not to be mistaken for an obstructed and dilated renal pelvis (**31**) (see page 50/61). The examiner should measure the diameter of the cyst and state its location (upper/lower pole or, respectively, upper, middle or lower third of the kidney), and should carefully look for tumorous lesions in its immediate vicinity. Some malignant renal tumors can contain cystic components that may be more conspicuous than the actual solid component of the tumor.

Finding a few renal cysts is clinically inconsequential, though re-evaluation at regular intervals is advisable. These simple renal cysts should be differentiated from the innumerable cysts (**64**) of the adult form of familial polycystic renal disease (**Fig. 46.3**). They show progressive growth and can reach a considerable size.

By displacing and thinning the renal parenchyma, polycystic renal disease leads to renal insufficiency in early adulthood and eventually to dialysis or renal transplant.

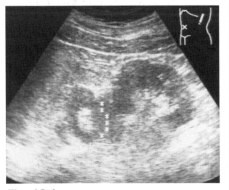

Fig. 46.1 a

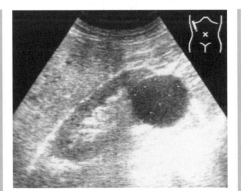

Fig. 46.2 a

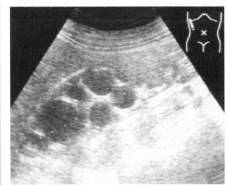

Fig. 46.3 a

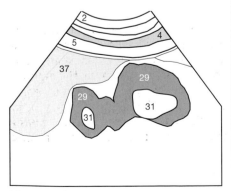

Fig. 46.1 b

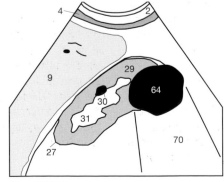

Fig. 46.2 b

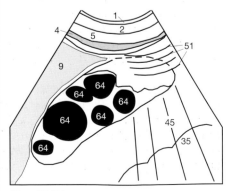

Fig. 46.3 b

The next two pages present the characteristic sonographic changes that play a special role in newborns and children and are different from the findings in adults.

Kidneys in Newborns

Before the kidneys are examined in the prone newborn (**Fig. 47.1a**), the urinary bladder should be examined supine, since the bladder can only be evaluated when it is full and newborns often void during the examination. Thereafter, the newborn is turned prone and both kidneys are scanned from the back with a 5.0 – 7.5 MHz linear transducer, longitudinally (**Fig. 47.1**) and transversely (**Fig. 47.2**). The transhepatic approach from the front (see page 45) or the lateroposterior approach in the lateral decubitus position is superior only in older infants.

With older children, lower center frequencies of 3.5 – 3.75 MHz are preferred. The normal measurements in childhood are stated as percentiles of the body size. A summary is found on page 51.

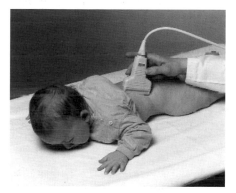

Fig. 47.1 a

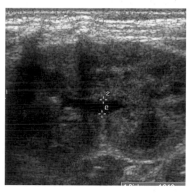

Fig. 47.1 b

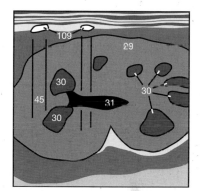

Fig. 47.1 c

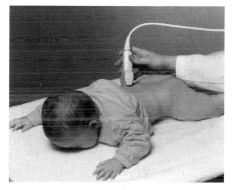

Fig. 47.2 a

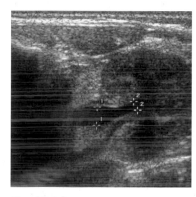

Fig. 47.2 b

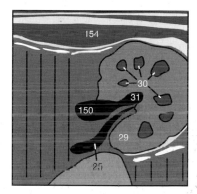

Fig. 47.2 c

Typical Variants in Newborns

In comparison to adult kidneys, the neonatal kidneys display a diffusely higher echogenicity of the parenchyma (**29**) with resultant pronounced demarcation of the hypoechoic medullary pyramids (**30**). Thus, the triangular shape of the medullary pyramids is better delineated than in adults, whose medullary pyramids appear more spherical.

Furthermore, many neonatal kidneys show a subtle fetal lobulation, which only resolves during infancy when the organ assumes a smooth, ovoid outline. The hyperechoic central complex of the pelvic region (**31**) appears just linear and thin in newborns, then increases gradually in width during infancy, attributed to the increasing deposition of fat between blood vessels and collecting system. Consequently, the anechoic pelvis is more conspicuous in newborn. It can measure up to 5 mm without indicating a urinary obstruction (see page 52).

The so-called dromedary hump, which refers to a thickened left lateral renal cortex opposite the inferior splenic border, is a typical renal configuration found in small infants and usually subsides with continuing organ growth. Hyperplastic columns of Bertini can traverse the hyperechoic pelvic region as hyperechoic parenchymal bridges, suggesting a renal duplication (compare with **Fig. 46.1**). Neither finding has a space-occupying effect and should not be mistaken for a renal tumor.

Diffusely Increased Echogenicity

While diffusely increased echogenicity of the renal parenchyma is normal in newborns (see preceding page), it becomes a sign of parenchymal damage in infants (**Fig. 48.1**). Equal or increased echogenicity of the renal parenchyma (**29**) is readily apparent in comparison to the liver (**9**) and especially to the medullary pyramids (**30**). Aside from glomerulonephritis and diffuse leukemic infiltration, possible causes include drug-induced damage, such as polychemotherapy, for example (**Fig. 48.2**), shown here together with early urinary tract obstruction (**31**).

Diffusely increased echogenicity of the kidney should prompt the examiner to search for pleural effusion (**Fig. 37.3**) or ascites in the lower pelvis (**Fig. 48.3**). Together with proteinuria and hypoproteinemia, this suggests a nephrotic syndrome. The example shown in **Figure 48.3** was intentionally selected to emphasize the risk of misinterpretation when the examination is performed after voiding. The urinary bladder is (**38**) is almost completely empty, so that the ascites (**68**) next to the small uterus (**39**) could have been incorrectly interpreted as the bladder.

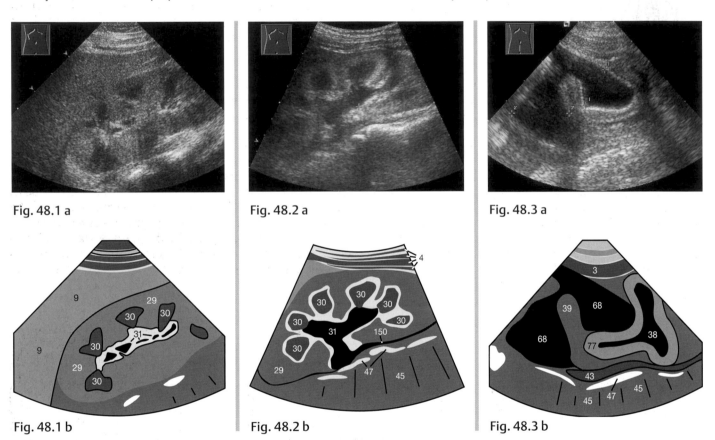

Fig. 48.1 a   Fig. 48.2 a   Fig. 48.3 a

Fig. 48.1 b   Fig. 48.2 b   Fig. 48.3 b

Nephrocalcinosis

The deposited crystals in nephrocalcinosis initially cause a hyperechoic scalloped rim around the medullary pyramids, with later hyperechoic extension to the caliceal apices or throughout the pyramids. Thus, the contrast is inverted, with hyperechoic medullary pyramids and a less echoic parenchymal rim. Initially, the calcifications do not show any acoustic shadowing.

The possible causes include tubular acidosis, urate nephropathy with massive cellular destruction as part of chemotherapy, vitamin D toxicity, and therapy with ACTH or furosemide. The diffusely hyperechoic medullary pyramid resembles the image found in a dehydrated newborn with precipitated proteins. After rehydration of the newborn, these precipitations of so-called Tamm-Horsfall proteins are reversible within a few days.

Nephritis

The kidney reacts to various inflammatory conditions with rather similar sonographic changes. In early pyelonephritis or glomerulonephritis, the kidney can appear entirely normal, but later edema enlarges its outline and interstitial infiltration enhances the parenchymal echogenicity with accentuated demarcation of the parenchyma (29) relative to the hypoechoic medullary pyramids (30) (Fig. 49.3). This is referred to as "punched-out medullary pyramids." Compared to the adjacent splenic or hepatic parenchyma (9), the parenchyma of the infiltrated kidney appears more hyperechoic (Fig. 49.3) than the parenchyma of the normal kidney (Fig. 46.3).

The increased echogenicity of the renal parenchyma does not permit any conclusion as to the nature of the inflammation. It can be found with interstitial nephritis, chronic glomerulonephritis, diabetic nephropathy, amyloidosis, autoimmune disease and urate nephropathy. The latter condition is caused by hyperuricemia as manifestation of gout or increased nucleic acid turnover. Sonography does not make an evidential contribution to the differential diagnosis between various inflammatory causes, but it plays a role in monitoring renal inflammation during therapy and excluding any complications. The resistive index (a measure of renal perfusion) determined by Doppler sonography can provide valuable information about the course of an infiltration or, for instance, an early rejection of a transplanted kidney. Inconclusive cases can benefit from sonography-guided percutaneous needle biopsy to obtain histologic confirmation.

In acute nephritis, the parenchyma can be diffusely hypoechoic and widened, and the junction between cortex and medulla can appear indistinct and washed out. Normal kidneys have a sharply demarcated corticomedullary junction.

Renal Atrophy

With increasing age, a slowly progressing decrease in the width of the parenchymal rim is physiologic (see page 45). A more pronounced atrophy of the parenchyma (Fig. 49.1) occurs after several inflammatory episodes or secondary to severe renal artery stenosis. Decreased perfusion either affects the entire kidney or is localized as infarcts, which are often embolic in nature (Fig. 54.3). In end-stage chronic nephritis, the markedly narrowed parenchyma (29) might be just barely sonographically detectable (Fig. 49.2). This illustrated example of an atrophic kidney shows the frequently accompanying finding of degenerative calcifications (53) or concrements (49), which are indirectly evident by their corresponding acoustic shadows (45). Atrophic kidneys can be so small that they elude sonographic detection.

The loss of excretory function in one kidney can be made up by compensatory hypertrophy of the contralateral kidney. In a unilaterally small kidney, the PPI (see page 45) should be determined first. A normal index suggests a developmentally hypoplastic kidney. In general, a diagnosis can be established by including the contralateral kidney in the examination and by evaluating the renal perfusion through color duplex sonography.

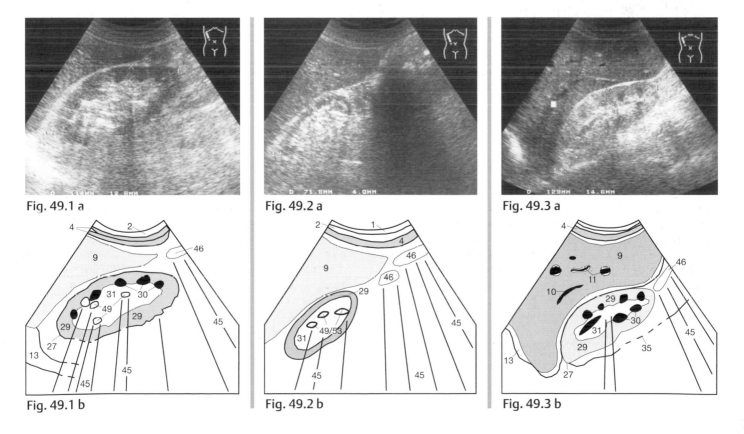

Fig. 49.1 a   Fig. 49.2 a   Fig. 49.3 a

Fig. 49.1 b   Fig. 49.2 b   Fig. 49.3 b

Normally, the collecting system is seen as a very hyperechoic central complex that is only traversed by thin, small vascular structures. With increased diuresis after intake of a large amount of fluid, the renal pelvis can distend and be seen as a anechoic structure (87) within the pelvic echo complex (31) (Fig. 50.1). The same finding can represent the developmental variant of an extrarenal pelvis. Either physiologic condition does not dilate the calices and infundibula.

Three degrees of urinary obstruction are distinguished in adults. The first degree of obstructive dilation distends the renal pelvis (87) but shows no infundibular extension or detectable parenchymal thinning (Fig. 50.2). The second degree of obstructive dilation causes additional fullness of the infundibula and calices (Fig. 50.3). In addition, a beginning parenchymal thinning might be detectable. The third degree of obstructive dilation is characterized by extensive pressure atrophy of the parenchyma.

Sonography cannot determine the possible causes of an obstructive uropathy in all cases. A ureteral stone is generally only visualized if it is lodged proximally at the ureteropelvic (UP) junction or distally in the prevesical ureter. The midureter is mostly obscured by overlying intestinal air. An exception is found in **Figure 50.4**, which shows a stone (49) in the ureter (150).

Less frequent causes of ureteral obstruction are tumors of the bladder or uterus and retroperitoneal fibrosis following radiation or idiopathic as manifestation of Ormond disease. Furthermore, aggregated lymph nodes can lead to ureteral compression. A latent obstruction can be caused by an atonic ureter in pregnancy, infections, and incomplete emptying of the bladder (neurogenic or secondary to prostatic hypertrophy, see page 73). In these cases, the sonographic evaluation must include measuring the post-void residual volume (see page 57).

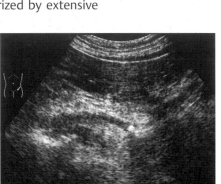

Fig. 50.4 a

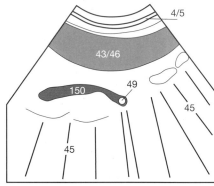

Fig. 50.4 b

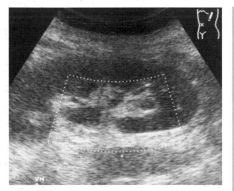

Fig. 50.1 a

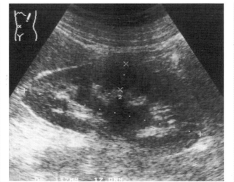

Fig. 50.2 a

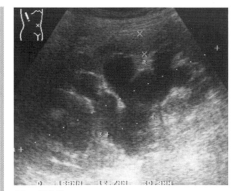

Fig. 50.3 a

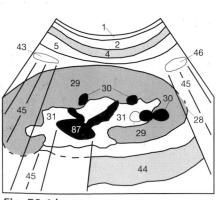

Fig. 50.1 b

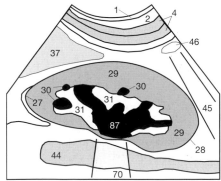

Fig. 50.2 b

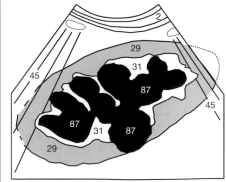

Fig. 50.3 b

Not every hypoechoic dilation of the renal pelvis (31) indicates a urinary obstruction. The developmental variant of an extrarenal pelvis was already mentioned on the preceding page. Furthermore, the renal hilum can show prominent vessels (25) (Fig. 51.1) that can be followed to the hypoechoic medullary pyramids (30) and mistaken for structures of the collecting system. These vessels generally appear rather delicate and lack the characteristic fullness of an obstructed and dilated collecting system (Fig. 50.2). The differential diagnosis can be easily solved by determining the flow with color-coded duplex sonography. With adequate setting, the blood flow is displayed as color while the static

or only slowly flowing urine remains black (= anechoic). The differentiation between a dilated collecting system (87) and parapelvic cysts (64) is more difficult (Fig. 51.2), especially if both conditions are present. Urinary obstruction in children is addressed on the pages 52 ff.

Alternative Methods

If sonography cannot solve the nature of a urinary obstruction, computed tomography (CT, Fig. 51.3) or the intravenous pyelogram (IVP, Fig. 51.4) can be turned to as other non-invasive methods. Either method can quantify the

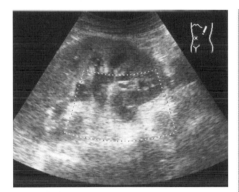

Fig. 51.1 a

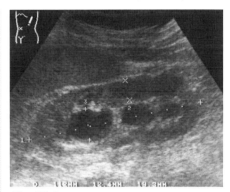

Fig. 51.2a

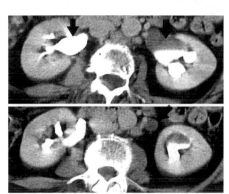

Fig. 51.3

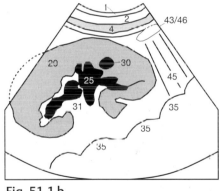

Fig. 51.1 b

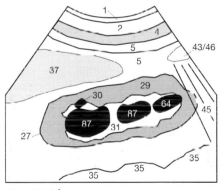

Fig. 51.2 b

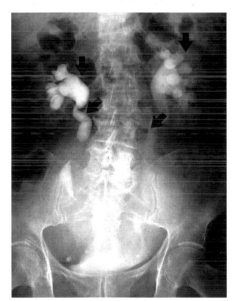

Fig. 51.4

Normal values of the kidneys in pediatrics
(For a German population, according to Dinkel E. et al.: Kidney Size in Childhood, Pediatr. Radiol. (15): 38-43)

Body size (cm)	$\overline{m} - 2\,SD$	$\overline{m}$	$\overline{m} + 2\,SD$
Newborns	3,40	4,16	4,92
< 55	3,00	4,35	5,83
55 – 70	3,60	5,00	6,40
71 – 85	4,50	5,90	7,30
86 – 100	5,30	6,60	7,90
101 – 110	5,85	7,10	8,35
111 – 120	6,35	7,65	8,95
121 – 130	6,90	7,20	9,50
131 – 140	7,40	8,70	10.00
141 – 150	7,90	9,25	10,60
> 150	8,60	9,95	11,30

dilation of both the intrarenal collecting system (↓) and the ureter (↙). Figures 51.3 and 51.4 belong to the same patient, who has caliceal clubbing that is more severe on the left than on the right and obstructive ureteral dilation.

P

To avoid any subsequent damage to the kidneys, a stenosis at the ureteropelvic junction or bladder orifice, as well as vesicoureteral reflux with resultant obstruction, should be detected with the first sonographic screening of a newborn.

It should be kept in mind that the delicate anechoic renal pelvis (31) can measure up to 5 mm wide (**Fig. 52.1**) in newborns without evidence of urinary obstruction. A renal pelvis measuring between 5 and 10 mm in width (**Fig. 52.2**) should be followed at short intervals to clarify whether it presents a congenital ampullary renal pelvis or a pathologic progressing dilation of the collecting system. Only a renal pelvis exceeding 10 mm in width (**Fig. 52.3**), clubbed calices (149) and a dilated ureter (150) are indications for an immediate diagnostic work-up (**Fig. 52.3**). A voiding cystourethrogram is generally performed (see next page).

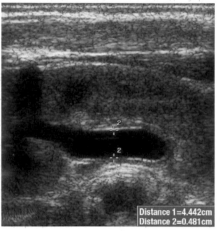

Fig. 52.1 a

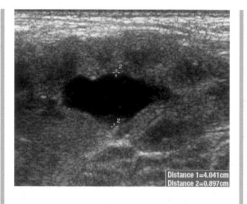

Fig. 52.2 a

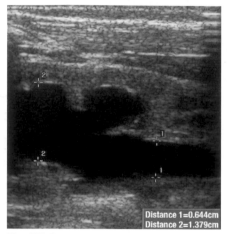

Fig. 52.3 a

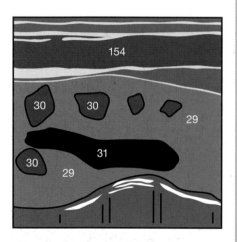

Fig. 52.1 b

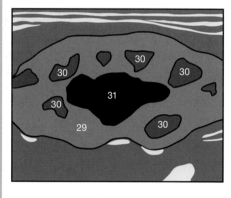

Fig. 52.2 b

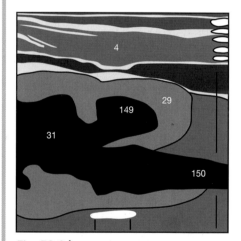

Fig. 52.3 b

If the ureter (150) is dilated in continuity with the renal pelvis (31) as seen in **Fig. 52.3**, a ureteropelvic stenosis can be excluded as cause of the urinary obstruction. An isolated dilation of the renal pelvis with or without caliceal clubbing should be further evaluated with a voiding cystourethrogram or intravenous pyelogram (IVP) to exclude vesicoureteral reflux or a ureteropelvic junction stenosis. The example shown in **Figure 52.3** shows a thinned parenchymal cortex due to urinary obstruction, indicative of immediate diagnostic work-up and possible decompression.

Width of the renal pelvis in newborns:

Normal	< 5 mm
Requiring follow up	5 - 10 mm
Suspicious for pathologic dilation	> 10 mm

Possible Sequelae of Urinary Obstruction

When urinary obstruction is not detected early, it can lead to thinning of the parenchymal cortex (**29** in **Fig. 53.1**) and gradually progress to renal atrophy (**Fig. 49.2**) with corresponding loss of renal function. Furthermore, chronic urinary tract infections or metabolic disturbances can induce crystalline precipitations (➤) in the dilated calices of the collecting system **(Fig. 53.2)**.

Grades of Reflux in Children

Grade I	Reflux into distal ureter
Grade II	Reflux into collecting system
Grade III	Additional beginning ureteral dilation and caliceal clubbing
Grade IV	More pronounced ureteral dilation and caliceal clubbing
Grade V	Marked caliceal clubbing and beginning parenchymal loss

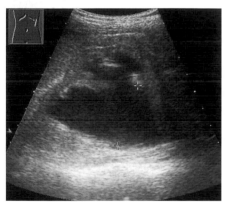

Fig. 53.1 a

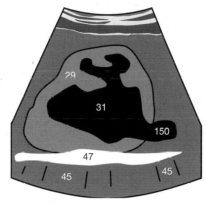

Fig. 53.1 b

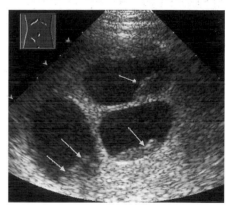

Fig. 53.2

Voiding Cystourethrogram

A voiding cystourethrogram excludes or detects vesicoureteral reflux and should be performed in patients with recurrent urinary tract infections or dilated collecting system in the infection-free interval after antibiotic therapy. Normally (**Fig. 53.3**), the completely filled urinary bladder shows no retrograde ureteral reflux (⟷) even during voiding as documented by contrast medium in the urethra (➡). The images are obtained with the patient slightly oblique to avoid mistaking the adjacent cortex of the ilium as grade I reflux (reflux into distal ureter only). A reflux into the collecting system (⬅) is called a grade II reflux **(Fig. 53.4)**. Additional dilation of the ureter and beginning clubbing of the calices indicate a grade III reflux.

Grade IV reflux refers to more pronounced caliceal clubbing and ureteral dilation, and grade V reflux to additional parenchymal scarring (see table). The chronic final stage is characterized by tortuosity of the entire dilated ureter as seen in **Fig. 53.5**.

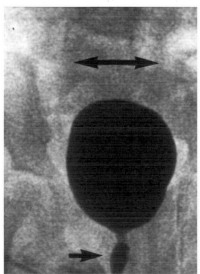
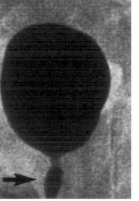

Fig. 53.3

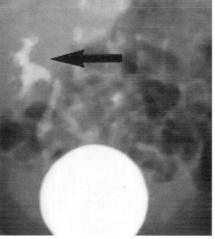

Fig. 53.4

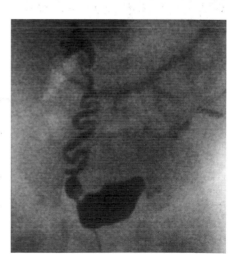

Fig. 53.5

Detecting concrements in the kidney (nephrolithiasis) is more difficult than detecting stones in the gallbladder (see page 42). The hyperechoic renal stones **(49)** often lie within the equally hyperechoic collecting system **(31)** (**Fig. 54.1**), and consequently are not discernible from their surrounding structures. Concrements in a dilated collecting system are a notable exception, since their echogenicity contrasts with the surrounding anechoic urine. The examiner must carefully search the hyperechoic collecting system for acoustic shadowing **(45)** cast by renal concrements or calcifications. **Figure 54.2** shows an example of extensive renal calcifications **(49)** in a patient with a markedly elevated serum calcium level as manifestation of hyperparathyroidism.

Depending on its composition, a renal stone **(49)** can be completely sound transmitting (**Fig. 54.1**) or so reflective that only its near surface is seen as hyperechoic cap (**Fig. 54.2**). The differential diagnosis includes arcuate arteries along the corticomedullary junction (bright echoes without shadowing), vascular calcifications in diabetic patients, and calcified fibrotic residues following renal tuberculosis. Papillary calcifications following phenacetin abuse is a rare differential diagnostic cause.

Large staghorn calculi are difficult to diagnose if the distal acoustic shadowing is weak and their hyperechogenicity is mistaken for the central hyperechoic complex.

Renal concrements can dislodge and migrate from the intrarenal collecting system into the ureter (**Fig. 50.4**). Depending on their size, they can pass into the bladder asymptomatically or with colic-like symptoms. Furthermore, they become lodged in the ureter and cause ureteral obstruction. In addition to detecting obstructive uropathy, sonography can exclude other causes of abdominal pain, such as pancreatitis, colitis and free fluid in the cul-de-sac (see page 58).

Renal Infarcts

Renal emboli arising from an aortic aneurysm (see page 21) or renal arterial stenosis can cause localized renal infarcts. Conforming to the vascular distribution, they are broad-based at the renal surface and tapered toward the renal hilus. Later, these triangular parenchymal defects **(71)** (**Fig. 54.3**) become hyperechoic scars. Considering their location and typical configuration, these hyperechoic scars should not be mistaken for renal concrements or tumors.

Besides digital substraction angiography (DSA), non-invasive color-coded duplex sonography is suitable for detecting renal artery stenosis. Especially difficult is the visualization and evaluation of small accessory renal arteries. They can arise as so-called upper or lower polar arteries from the aorta in the immediate vicinity or at some distance from the major renal artery or, in rare instances, from the common iliac artery.

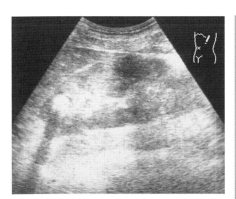

Fig. 54.1 a

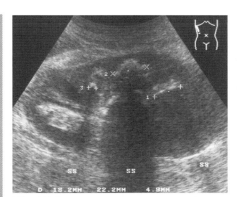

Fig. 54.2 a

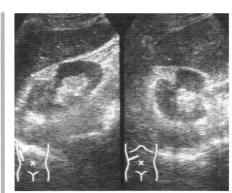

Fig. 54.3 a

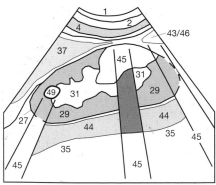

Fig. 54.1 b

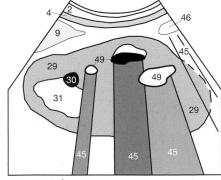

Fig. 54.2 b

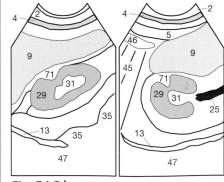

Fig. 54.3 b

Solid renal tumors differ from fluid-filled cysts by internal echoes and no or only weak distal acoustic enhancement.

Benign Renal Tumors

Solid benign renal tumors (fibromas, adenomas and hemangiomas) are altogether rare and show a variegated sonographic morphology. Only the angiomyolipoma, a benign mixed tumor comprising vessels, muscular tissue and fat, has in its early stage a characteristic sonographic presentation that separates it from a malignant process. A small angiomyolipoma (72) is as hyperechoic as the central echo complex (31) and clearly demarcated (Fig. 55.1). Sonographically, it is similar to the hepatic hemangioma (Figs. 37.2 and 37.3). With increasing size, the angiomyolipomas become heterogeneous, rendering their differentiation from malignant tumors more difficult.

Malignant Renal Tumors

Small renal cell carcinomas (54) are often isoechoic with the remaining renal parenchyma (29). Only with further growth do they become more heterogeneous and space-occupying, with bulging of the renal contour (Fig. 55.2). If a carcinoma has been detected, both renal veins and the inferior vena cava have to be carefully scrutinized for tumor tissue because of the known tendency of intravenous tumorous extension. Renal cell carcinomas can be bilateral in about 5% of cases. If the tumor extends beyond the renal capsule and infiltrates the surrounding tissue, the kidney loses its physiologic respiratory mobility (see page 45). Finally, portions of malignant renal tumors can contain cystic areas, and benign-appearing renal cysts should always be evaluated for space-occupying solid lesions in their vicinity.

Tumors of the Adrenal Gland

The left adrenal gland lies anteromedial (not superior) to the upper renal pole. The right adrenal gland usually lies somewhat superior to the upper pole of the right kidney and posterior to the inferior vena cava. In adults, both adrenal glands are not at all or only barely visible in the perirenal fat. This does not apply to the adrenal glands in newborns (see page 56).

Hormone-producing adrenal tumors, such as adenomas in Conn syndrome or hyperplasia in Cushing syndrome, are generally too small to be detectable sonographically. Only clinically manifest pheochromocytomas have often reached several centimeters in size and 90% can be sonographically detected. Inconclusive cases should be further evaluated by CT.

Sonography plays a more important role in the detection of adrenal metastases (54), which are usually seen as hypoechoic lesions (Fig. 55.3) between upper renal pole and spleen (37) or inferior hepatic surface, respectively. They must be differentiated from superficial renal cysts. The exquisite vascularity of the adrenal glands explains the hematogenous spread of metastases from carcinomas of the lung, breast and kidney. The echogenicity of a suprarenal lesion does not allow a reliable conclusion of its histologic nature or a differentiation from a neurinoma arising from the sympathetic chain.

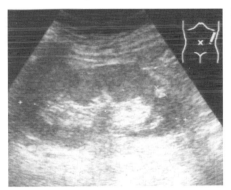

Fig. 55.1 a

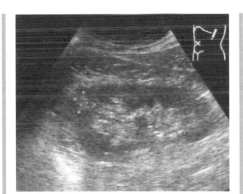

Fig. 55.2 a

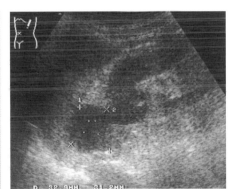

Fig. 55.3 a

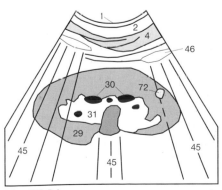

Fig. 55.1 b

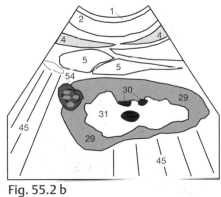

Fig. 55.2 b

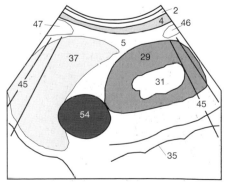

Fig. 55.3 b

Benign Renal Tumors

Aside from fibromas as manifestation of neurofibromatosis (Recklinghausen disease), benign space-occupying lesions of the pediatric kidney include angiomyolipomas, which occur together with Bourneville-Pringle disease (tuberous sclerosis) and resemble angiomyolipomas found in adults (**Fig. 55.1**).

Nephroblastoma

The nephroblastoma (**54**) is the most frequent malignant space-occupying lesion in the pediatric age group (**Figs. 56.1** and **56.2**). This tumor, also referred to as Wilms tumor, leads to a complete destruction of the normal renal anatomy and frequently shows a heterogeneous, hyperechoic internal structure with impaired urinary drainage from the remaining parenchyma (**29**), as shown in **Figure 56.3**. It is important to examine the contralateral kidney to exclude bilateral renal involvement, which has been observed in up to 10% of cases.

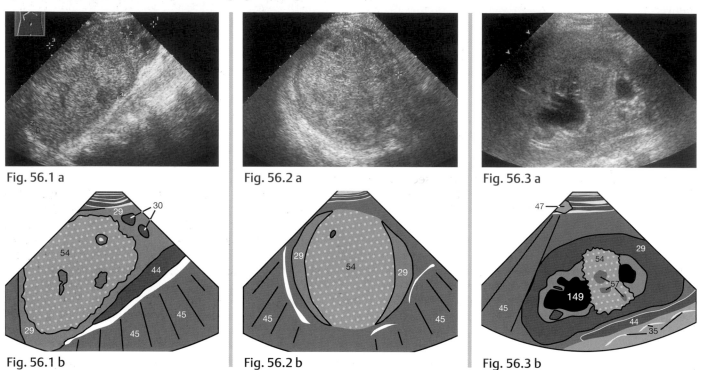

Fig. 56.1 a Fig. 56.2 a Fig. 56.3 a

Fig. 56.1 b Fig. 56.2 b Fig. 56.3 b

Lymphomatous Infiltration and Metastases

Less common are lymphomatous or metastatic infiltrations of the kidneys. Since the difference in echogenicity between involved areas and normal renal parenchyma (**29**) may not be very conspicuous (**Fig. 56.3**), such lesions often become only visible by central necroses (**57**) or associated urinary obstruction of adjacent caliceal groups (**149**).

Adrenal Glands

In newborns, the hypoechoic cortex of the adrenal gland can invariably be distinguished from the hyperechoic medulla (**155**) (**Fig. 56.4**). Seen from posterior, the adrenal gland usually shows a typical Y-shape superolaterally to the upper renal pole. This difference in echogenicity disappears during infancy and the adult adrenal glands are barely separable from perirenal fat (**Fig. 49.1**).

In newborns, bleeding in the adrenal glands usually presents as hypoechoic area (↘) at the upper renal pole (**Fig. 56.5**). If this finding is indeed a hematoma, it should measurably decrease in size within a month. If its size is unchanged, a cystic neuroblastoma must be excluded through laboratory parameters or MRI. Adenomas of the adrenal gland are less common and, because of their small size, can often be detected solely by high-resolution CT with density measurements of the unenhanced images.

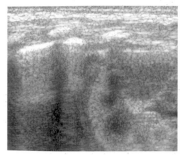

Fig. 56.4 a

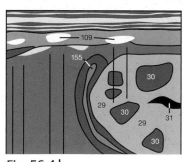

Fig. 56.4 b

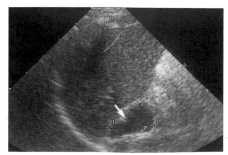

Fig. 56.5

Examination Protocol

The urinary bladder is systematically scanned in suprapubical transverse (**Fig. 57.1a**) and longitudinal (**Fig. 57.1b**) sections. Only by moving the transducer slowly can the examiner detect suspicious wall thickening or intraluminal lesions. It has been found useful to include the adjacent lateral perivesical tissue. If possible, the bladder should be maximally filled after drinking a large amount of clear

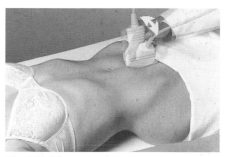

Fig. 57.1 a

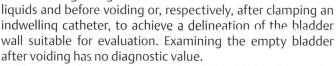

Fig. 57.1 b

liquids and before voiding or, respectively, after clamping an indwelling catheter, to achieve a delineation of the bladder wall suitable for evaluation. Examining the empty bladder after voiding has no diagnostic value.

The typical transverse section (**Fig. 57.2**) shows the normal urinary bladder (**38**) behind both rectal muscles (**3**) and above and behind the rectum (**43**). If filled to capacity, the bladder exhibits the configuration of a rectangle with rounded corners. On the sagittal longitudinal section (**Fig. 57.3**), the urinary bladder appears more triangular. Inferior to the urinary bladder, the prostate gland (**42**) or vagina can be visualized (**Figs. 73.2** and **75.1**).

Measuring the Postvoid Residual

If neurogenic dysfunction or obstruction due to hypertrophy of the prostate gland (see page 73) is suspected, the bladder volume should be calculated for determining the postvoid residual. The greatest transverse diameter (**Fig. 57.2b**) is

taken from the transverse section and the greatest supero-inferior diameter from the sagittal section (the horizontal dotted line in **Fig. 57.3b**). To obtain a suitable sagittal section, it is often necessary to rock the transducer caudally as shown in **Figure 57.3a** to work around any interfering acoustic shadowing (**45**) of the pubic bone (**48**). The greatest anteroposterior diameter (vertically dotted line in both shown sonographic images) can be taken from either image plane.

The postvoid residual can be calculated in ml using the simplified volume formula of the product of the three diameters multiplied by 0.5. Even though a postvoid residual up to 100 ml has been stated in the literature as still physiologic, a bladder outlet obstruction should be considered if the postvoid residual is calculated to be more than 50 ml.

Volume determination of the urinary bladder
Volume = A x B x C x 0.5

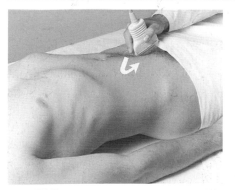

Fig. 57.2 a

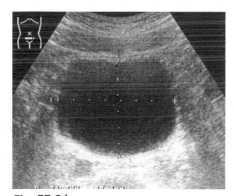

Fig. 57.2 b

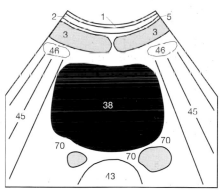

Fig. 57.2 c

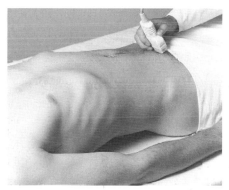

Fig. 57.3 a

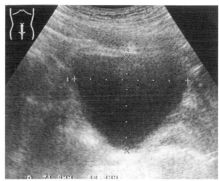

Fig. 57.3 b

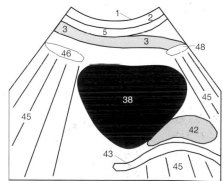

Fig. 57.3 c

The urinary bladder **(38)** with an indwelling catheter **(76)** is usually collapsed and consequently cannot be adequately evaluated. It is therefore necessary to clamp the catheter some time before the examination (think of it!) to fill the urinary bladder. Only a rather advanced edema of the bladder wall **(77)** can be considered diagnostic of cystitis **(Fig. 58.2)**, even with the bladder empty. The wall thickness of a distended (filled) urinary bladder should not exceed 4 mm. After voiding, even the normal urinary bladder wall is irregular and up to 8 mm thick, potentially masking wall-based polyps or localized tumors.

Wall Thickening

Diffuse wall thickening involving the entire circumference is mostly edematous as manifestation of cystitis. Localized wall thickening is more suspicious for a wall-based tumor. The differential diagnosis must consider trabeculations compensating a bladder outlet obstruction due to prostatic hypertrophy. In inconclusive cases, transrectal endosonography with higher frequencies or CT might clarify the situation.

Internal Echoes and Sedimentations

Even the healthy bladder is never entirely anechoic (= black). The bladder **(38)** often shows reverberation artifacts **(51a)** induced by the anterior abdominal wall **(Fig. 58.3)** in its lumen near the transducer. In the posterior bladder lumen away from the transducer, section thickness artifacts **(51b)** are often observed, caused by the oblique course of the bladder wall relative to the sound beam. They can also simulate intraluminal matter (see page 14). These artifacts have to be differentiated from true sedimentations of crystals, small

blood clots **(52)** or concrements **(49)** along the floor of the urinary bladder **(Fig. 58.3)**. By rapidly changing the pressure applied to the transducer (be careful with an overdistended bladder...), intraluminal matter can be shaken up and made to float within the lumen. Of course, a wall-based tumor does not respond to this maneuver.

Ureter Peristalsis

Incidental evidence of propulsive ureter peristalsis can often be observed as a jet of urine propelled from the ureteral ostium into the bladder lumen. Furthermore, ureteroceles must be excluded in infants **(Fig. 59.4)**.

Free Fluid

In any abdominal trauma, it is essential to detect or exclude free fluid **(68)** in the abdomen. **Figure 58.4** shows free fluid in its typical location in the cul-de-sac behind the uterus **(39)**, as found, for example, in acute intra-abdominal bleeding.

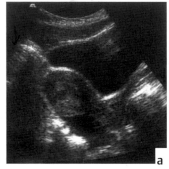
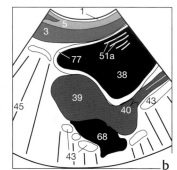

Fig. 58.4

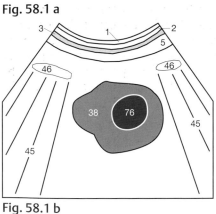

Fig. 58.1 a

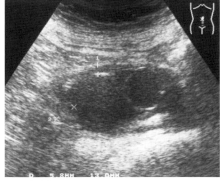

Fig. 58.2 a

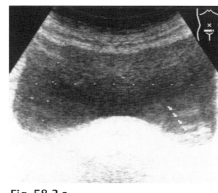

Fig. 58.3 a

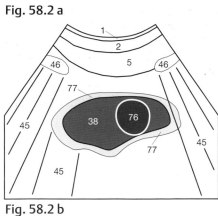

Fig. 58.1 b

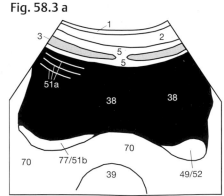

Fig. 58.2 b

Fig. 58.3 b

Urachal Duct

In the newborn, the bladder is best examined with suprapubic longitudinal and transverse sections (**Fig. 59.1a**), as long as the bladder is filled (this means at the beginning of the examination!). Special attention should be given to the bladder roof (**Fig. 59.1b**) to check for a persistent urachal canal, which appears as hypoechoic tubular structure (↖) along the anterior abdominal wall between umbilicus (↑) and bladder roof (**Fig. 59.2**).

Hematoma and Cystitis

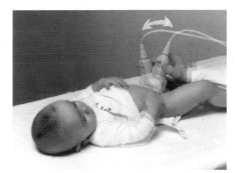

Fig. 59.1 a

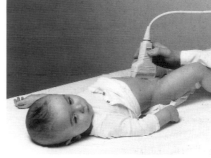

Fig. 59.1 b

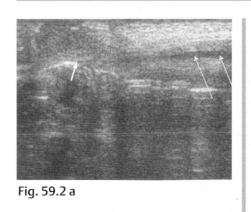

Fig. 59.2 a

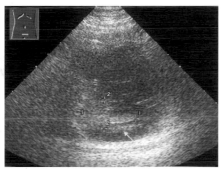

Fig. 59.3 a

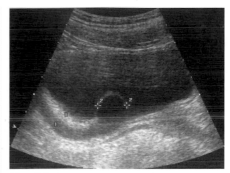

Fig. 59.4 a

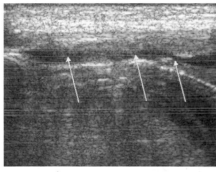

Fig. 59.2 b

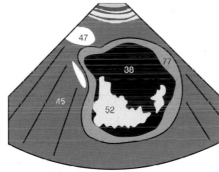

Fig. 59.3 b

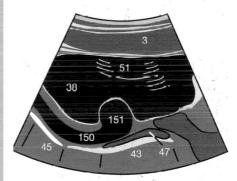

Fig. 59.4 b

In children, the most common space-occupying lesions in the urinary bladder (**38**) are blood clots (**52**), which are usually the result of a hemorrhagic cystitis (**Fig. 59.3**). This child received chemotherapy in preparation for a bone marrow transplant. As in adults (**Fig. 58.2**), a cystitis manifests itself as wall thickening (**77**).

Ureterocele

In infants presenting with urinary obstruction, a uterocele (**151**) should be excluded besides a ureteral obstruction at the UP junction or ostium. A ureterocele can bulge into the bladder lumen as a thin membranous structure (**Fig. 59.4**), which may change in size and shape depending on the degree of filling. The case illustrated here also shows the dilated distal ureter (**150**).

Renal transplants can be located in either iliac fossa and are connected to the iliac vessels. Like the orthotopic kidneys, they are sonographically examined in two planes (**Fig. 60.1**), but the transducer is placed over the lateral aspect of the lower abdomen with the patient supine. Interfering intestinal air is absent because of the superficial position of the transplanted kidney just beneath the anterior abdominal wall. This location makes sonographic follow-up easy.

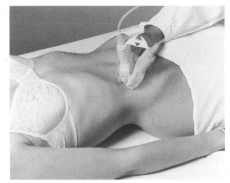 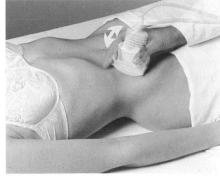

Fig. 60.1 a

Fig. 60.1 b

Normal Appearance of Renal Transplants

The normal renal transplant shows an often permanent increase in size by up to 20%. Compared to the native kidneys, its cortex (**29**) appears wider (**Fig. 60.2**) and the parenchymal echogenicity can be heightened with more conspicuous medullary pyramids (**30**) in comparison to native kidneys. Initially, serial sonographic studies should be obtained at short intervals to exclude a progressing inflammatory infiltration. A prominent renal pelvis or low-grade urinary distension (**Figs. 50.1** and **50.2**) might be observed without functional impairment of the renal transplant in need of intervention. The urinary distension should be documented and its cross-section measured (**Fig. 60.3**) to avoid missing any progression requiring therapeutic intervention on subsequent studies.

Early Detection of Rejection

The renal transplant should be further evaluated for a distinctive outline against surrounding tissues and a distinctive interface between parenchyma (**29**) and collecting system (**31**). A blurry interface or a slightly increased volume can be warning signs of a beginning rejection. For a valid comparison with subsequent studies, reproducible longitudinal and transverse diameters should be measured and documented (see page 61). Furthermore, the resistive index (RI) of the renal vessels determined by Doppler sonography should provide a valuable marker of early rejection. With increasing time after the implantation, immunosuppressive medications can be reduced and the intervals between serial sonographic studies extended.

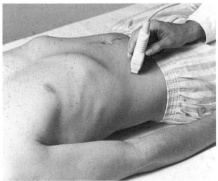 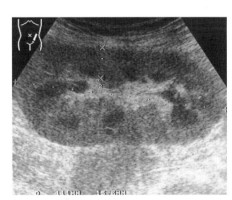 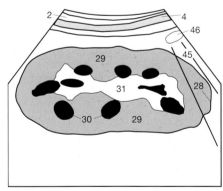

Fig. 60.2 a

Fig. 60.2 b

Fig. 60.2 c

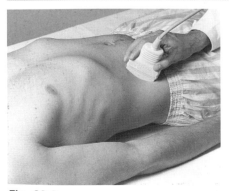 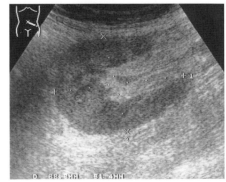 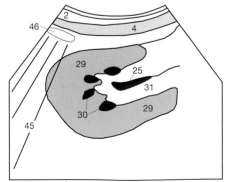

Fig. 60.3 a

Fig. 60.3 b

Fig. 60.3 c

For accurate assessment of its size, the renal transplant has to be scanned longitudinally **(Fig. 61.1b)** until the maximal length comes into view. The diagram **(Fig. 61.1a)** illustrates a line drawn too far laterally (dotted line) that would measure a spuriously short distance. The transducer must be moved following the straight arrows to measure the true longitudinal dimension (d_L).

Thereafter, the transducer is slightly rotated **(Fig. 61.1c)** to assure that the renal transplant has not been sectioned obliquely, as indicated by the second dotted black line in **Figure 61.1a**. The angulation has to be eliminated by rotating the transducer along the curved arrow. This two-step approach to guiding the transducer should assure that the documented length is not too short, which could lead to the misdiagnosis of a rejection due to a spuriously increased volume on follow-up examinations.

Lymphocele

A lymphocele **(73)** can develop as complication after renal transplant surgery **(Fig. 61.2)** and is usually found between the lower pole of the renal transplant **(29)** and the urinary bladder **(38)**, but can be anywhere adjacent to the renal transplant. Not every lymphocele requires an intervention. Small lymphoceles often resolve spontaneously. On first sight, large lymphoceles can occasionally be mistaken for the urinary bladder.

Urinary Obstruction

Urinary obstruction **(87)** is an equally frequent postoperative complication caused by reimplantation of the ureter. Depending on its severity, it might require temporary stent drainage **(59)** **(Figs. 61.3** and **61.4)** to prevent damage of the renal parenchyma **(29)**.

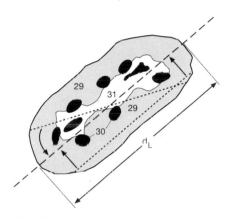

Fig. 61.1 a

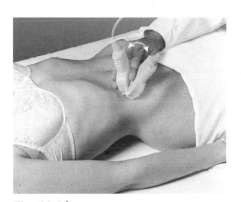

Fig. 61.1 b

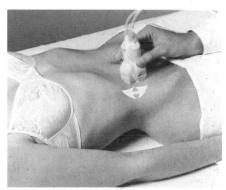

Fig. 61.1 c

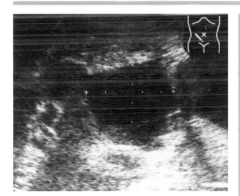

Fig. 61.2 a

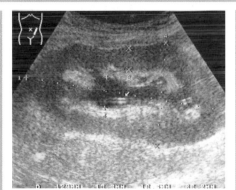

Fig. 61.3 a

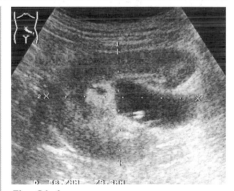

Fig. 61.4 a

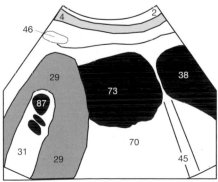

Fig. 61.2 b

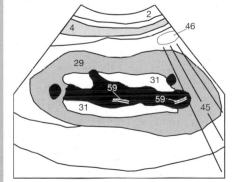

Fig. 61.3 b

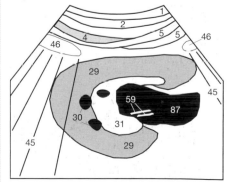

Fig. 61.4 b

This quiz should just help you to test your knowledge, clarify your understanding or fill gaps before you move on to the next organ system. Use it in the spirit of self-improvement and you will enjoy this quiz. You find the answers on the preceding pages (questions 1 to 5 and 8) or on page 108 (image questions 6, 7, 9).

1. From memory, draw a typical transverse section of the right kidney and pay attention to the medullary pyramids relative to the junction between the parenchyma and collecting system (maximum 2 minutes). Repeat this task for a transverse section of the right kidney at the level of its hilum, and consider its position relative to the liver and the inferior vena cava. Repeat both tasks (important: with breaks longer than 2 hours) until you accomplish them error-free.

2. Try to sketch the different shapes of the normal kidney in comparison with the corresponding images for a urinary obstruction, grade I to III. Discuss the differentiating criteria with a fellow student. Validate your sketches by comparing them with the images on pages 49/50.

3. How do you recognize nephrolithiasis? What are a few possible underlying conditions? With the help of material taken from the literature, provide a differential diagnosis of hematuria (blood in the urine).

4. List the sonographic criteria of a renal angiomyolipoma. What type of tumor is this? Why can it be difficult to differentiate it from other tumor types?

5. Do you remember the normal values for the renal size, the parenchyma-pelvis index (PPI) and the grades of urinary obstruction in children and adults? Write down your values and compare them with those listed on pages 45 and 51, 53.

6. Carefully review the sonographic images in **Figures 62.1** and **62.2** and write down the imaging planes, all visualized organs, vessels and muscles – and, of course, your working diagnosis and your reasoning behind it.

Questions with emphasis on pediatrics:

7. **Figure 62.3** is a voiding cystourethrogram (conventional radiographic view) of a child's pelvis at the time of voiding. Please look closely and give your diagnosis.

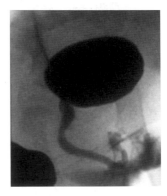

Fig. 62.3

8. How wide can the normal collecting system measure in a term newborn? At how many mm in pelvic width do you ask for a follow-up study or additional measures to exclude a urinary obstruction?

9. This image **(Fig. 62.4)** shows a transverse section of the upper abdomen at the level of the renal vessels. Describe the organs and vessels that you can recognize. Which vessel is atypical in its course and what conclusion do you draw from that?

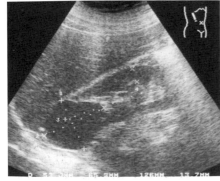

Fig. 62.1

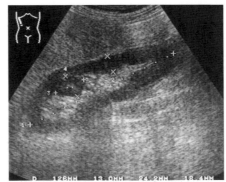

Fig. 62.2

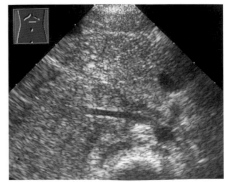

Fig. 62.4

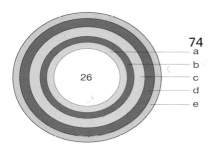

Fig. 63.1:
Mural layers of the stomach (74)
a   Mucosa:
    Epithelium + tunica propria
b   Muscularis mucosae
c   Submucosa
d   Muscular layer
    (longitudinal and circular muscles)
e   Serosa

The normal mural layering of the gastrointestinal (GI) tract consists of five layers, which appear alternatively hyperechoic and hypoechoic **(Fig. 63.1)**. The two hypoechoic layers correspond to the muscularis mucosa **(74b)** and to the somewhat thicker tunica muscularis **(74d)**. If the sound conditions are good or the stomach is filled with water or collapsed **(26)**, all mural layers **(74a-e)** can be identified **(Fig. 63.2)**. The outer serosal surface **(74e)** merges anteriorly with the also hyperechoic capsule of the liver **(9)** and, depending on the echogenicity of the adjacent pancreas **(33)**, is not always discernible posteriorly.

Depending on its state of contraction, the width of the gastric wall in adults varies between 5 and 7 mm. The hypoechoic tunica muscularis by itself should not measure more than 5 mm, unless a peristaltic wave passes through it **(Fig. 63.3)**. Occasionally, acoustic shadowing **(45)** of gastric air **(47)** can preclude the visualization of the posterior gastric wall. In pediatrics, the hypoechoic muscularis of a term newborn should not exceed 4 mm through the end of second month of life. The entire diameter of the pylorus should measure less than 15 mm. Hypertrophic pyloric stenosis is present whenever the cross-sectional diameter **(Fig. 63.4)** exceeds these values or the pylorus measures more than 16 mm in length (in this case about 22 mm) on the longitudinal section **(Fig. 63.5)**.

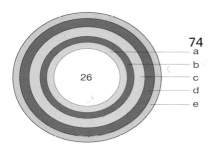

Fig. 63.2 a

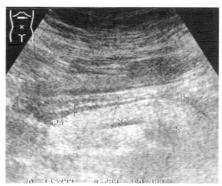

Fig. 63.2 b

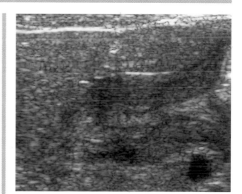

Fig. 63.2 c

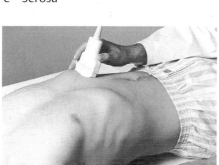

Fig. 63.3 a

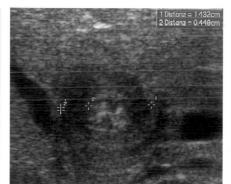

Fig. 63.4 a

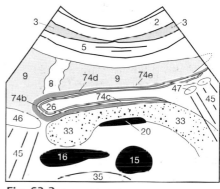

Fig. 63.5 a

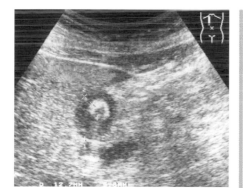

Fig. 63.3 b

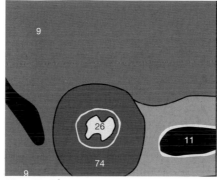

Fig. 63.4 b

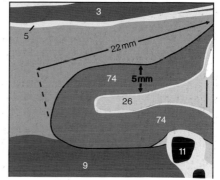

Fig. 63.5 b

P

Gastroesophageal Reflux

To confirm an insufficient lower esophageal sphincter with esophageal reflux in children, the child should be examined with the stomach filled after drinking a small amount of fluid or, if it is a newborn, after nursing. In either case, the swallowed fluid invariably contains air bubbles **(47)** and can be visualized as hyperechoic motion within the stomach **(26)**, often with comet tails or acoustic shadows **(45)** **(Fig. 64.1)**. After placing the esophageal hiatus of the diaphragm into the right sagittal longitudinal image plane **(Fig. 19.2)**, the esophagus will be observed for some time, possibly with the patient in the head-down position, to see whether gastric content refluxes across the distal sphincter into the esophagus. In adults, it is preferable to perform pulsed fluoroscopy after ingestion of an oral contrast medium.

Gastric Tumors

Depending on their histology, focal tumors can invade the normal mural layers (see preceding page). A dilated lumen **(26)** can be found as an indirect sign of a tumor-induced delay in gastric emptying **(Fig. 64.2)**. In this case, the delayed gastric emptying was caused by a large wall-based tumor **(54)** that had invaded the normal mural layers and almost completely blocked the lumen.

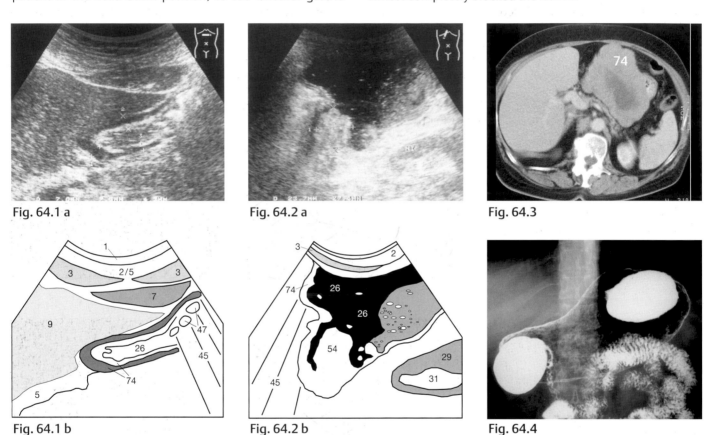

Fig. 64.1 a

Fig. 64.2 a

Fig. 64.3

Fig. 64.1 b

Fig. 64.2 b

Fig. 64.4

Alternative Imaging Modalities

Since intragastric air often leads to a sonographically incomplete visualization of the stomach, other diagnostic modalities are often applied.

Computed Tomography (CT)

The advantage of CT is its superiority in identifying any thickening of the gastric mural layers **(74)**, as in the diffuse lymphomatous infiltration of the stomach shown in **Figure 64.3**. Furthermore, CT can define any infiltration of regional lymph nodes and other neighboring organs better, regardless of the amount of air in the gastrointestinal tract. However, invasive gastroscopy is still needed to determine the histology of the tumor.

Upper GI Series

An upper GI series with double contrast visualization of the stomach is performed with the patient NPO to achieve good mucosal coating with the contrast medium (barium sulfate or water-soluble Gastrografin®). Together with the contrast medium, the patient takes an effervescent powder that releases CO_2 when it comes into contact with water. Next, the patient turns once or twice on the examination table. The released CO_2 distends the stomach and the gastric mucosal pattern can be fluoroscopically searched for lesions, rigid mural segments or ulcer craters **(Fig. 64.4)**. Do you know the position of this patient with a normal finding? Left or right lateral decubitus, supine or Trendelenburg position? The patient's position is revealed by the distribution of contrast medium. The answer is found on page 109.

Small bowel loops are rarely visualized because of the normally thin intestinal walls and are only noted by the acoustic shadowing of intestinal air. In inflammatory conditions, however, the wall becomes thickened at the expense of the intestinal lumen, rendering the wall considerably more conspicuous. Sonography has the advantage of real-time observation of the dynamics of intestinal peristalsis. The patient observer should be able to identify atonic segments (lacking peristalsis) or prestenotic hyperperistalsis.

Crohn's Disease

This disease frequently affects the terminal ileum (terminal ileitis). The involved intestinal segment shows edematous wall thickening (74) and becomes easily separable from adjacent uninvolved loops (46) (Fig. 65.1). Advanced stages can cause such a massively thickened intestinal wall (Fig. 65.2) that its sonographic cross-section is easily misinterpreted as a tumorous space-occupying lesion or mistaken for an intestinal invagination (see page 66). The terms "cockade phenomenon" and "target sign," which refer to the concentric lamellation of the thickened edematous wall, have been applied to this finding. Its surroundings and the cul-de-sac (Fig. 58.4) should always be searched for free intra-abdominal fluid as evidence of a perforation. Long segments of mural thickening are not only induced by an inflammation, but can also represent diffuse lymphomatous infiltration of the intestine, which is primarily found in immunosuppressed patients.

Ascites

The mesenteric roots of individual small bowel loops are normally not identifiable, but can be delineated in the presence of extensive lymphadenopathy or massive ascites (Fig. 65.3). The cross-sectionally displayed small bowel loop here (46) floats within ascitic fluid (68), which is devoid of internal echoes (hemorrhage?) except for reverberation artifacts (51) from the anterior abdominal wall (2, 3).

Hernias

The protrusion of an intestinal loop (46) through the anterior abdominal fasciae (6) is frequently observed around the umbilicus (Fig. 65.4) and along the linea alba. The size of the defect (◄—►) determines the risk of incarceration. A large defect is less likely to press on the vessels supplying the herniated intestinal loop (120). Ischemic thickening of the herniated intestinal loop (74) (not present here) should be looked for as an indirect sign of hypoperfusion.

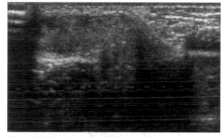

Fig. 65.4 a

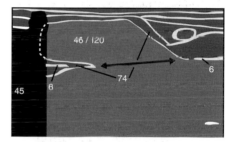

Fig. 65.4 b

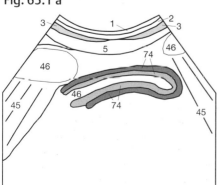

Fig. 65.1 a

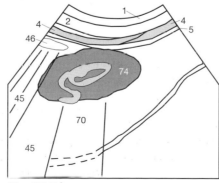

Fig. 65.2 a

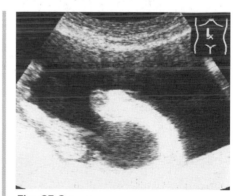

Fig. 65.3 a

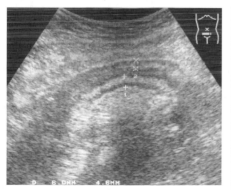

Fig. 65.1 b

Fig. 65.2 b

Fig. 65.3 b

Intussusception

The preferred age for an intussusception in the newborn is the sixth to ninth month. Males are more frequently affected than females. As a rule of thumb, an intussusception is a rarity, i.e., quite unlikely, before the third month and after the third year. The patient typically has pain episodes of abrupt onset with little or no pain in between. Usually, the terminal ileum protrudes through the ileocecal valve into the colon, causing a circular intestinal wall to be within the colonic lumen (**Figs. 66.1** and **66.2**). Intussusceptions involving the jejunum are rare.

The intussusception produces an external hypoechoic muscular layer (**74d**) separated from the internal invaginated muscularis by the hyperechoic mucosa (**74b**). Its cross-section shows concentric rings, referred to as target or bull's eye sign. Occasionally, even two echogenic mucosal layers (**74b**) of both intestinal segments are discernible (**Fig. 66.2**). **Figure 66.3** shows a CT with the findings of an intussusception (**74**), shown here next to air-containing colon segments (**43**).

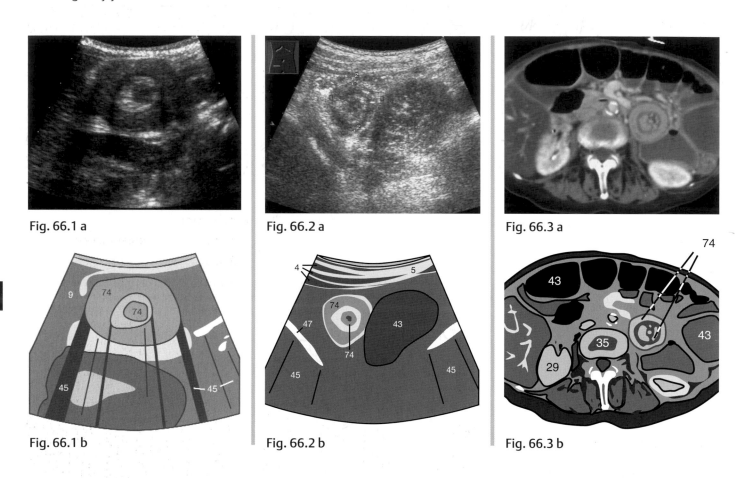

Fig. 66.1 a

Fig. 66.2 a

Fig. 66.3 a

Fig. 66.1 b

Fig. 66.2 b

Fig. 66.3 b

Contrast Enema

Whenever an intussusception has been confirmed by either method, the reduction of the intussuscepted intestinal segment (↘) should be immediately attempted by means of a contrast enema (**Fig. 66.4**). This is neccessary in order to prevent or resolve a vascular compression of the involved mesenteric root. In this case, the intussuscepted intestinal segment had already reached the mid transverse colon.

Ideally, the hydrostatic pressure of the retrograde instilled contrast medium completely pushes back the intussuscepted intestinal segment, thus avoiding a surgical intervention. The sonographic confirmation of the reposition is important. A concentric ring formation should no longer be visible. Occasionally, the intussusception recurs after successful reposition, which must be treated by a repeat contrast enema or by surgery.

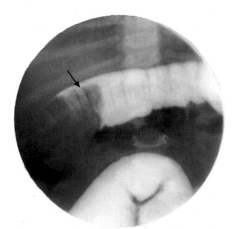

Fig. 66.4

Appendicitis

The normal appendix has a hyperechoic layer surrounded by a hypoechoic layer (**Fig. 67.1**). The maximal diameter of a normal appendix should not measure more than 6 mm and the mural layer not more than 2 mm. Measurements of 7 mm and 3 mm or more, respectively, are pathologic.

In addition, an acute appendicitis typically causes edematous mural thickening, which appears as a hypoechoic ring with a hyperechoic center (mucosa and narrowed lumen) on cross section (**Fig. 67.2a**). On longitudinal section (**Fig. 67.2b**), the appendix cannot be mistaken for another intestinal structure by lack of peristalsis and its blind end. In addition, local tenderness can be tested by applying gentle pressure on the transducer. The perifocal intestinal loops can show reactively reduced peristalsis. An abscess presents as an increasingly heterogenous and hyperechoic conglomeration that in its late stage is difficult to identify as an appendix.

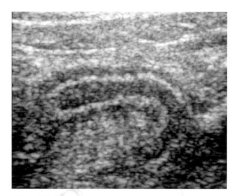

Fig. 67.1

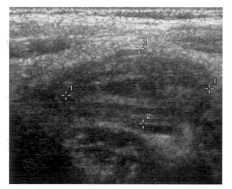

Fig. 67.2 a

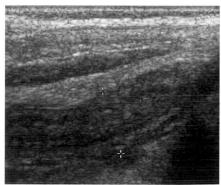

Fig. 67.2 b

Diarrhea

In watery diarrhea, a large amount of anechoic fluid (46) is found in the intestinal loops (**Fig. 67.3**). These intraluminal fluid accumulations should not be mistaken for extraluminal ascites (**Fig. 65.3**). The intestinal content is more echogenic in coprostasis (**Fig. 68.1**) or Hirschsprung disease.

Hirschsprung Disease

The megacolon of Hirschsprung disease is characterized by an aganglionic and resulting narrowed lumen with a massive dilation of the proximal colon segment (43), which has a luminal width clearly different from adjacent intestinal loops (46) (**Fig. 67.4**).

Familial clustering involves boys in about 80% of cases. A typical funnel-shaped transition is found from the narrowed segment to the megacolon. Frequently, the dilated lumen only contains little intestinal air (47) with posterior acoustic shadowing (45), permitting good sound transmission through the retained fecal matter.

Appendix, Normal Values		
	Normal	Inflammatory
Wall thickness	≤ 2 mm	≥ 3 mm
Maximal external diameter	< 6 mm	≥ 7 mm

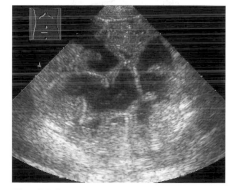

Fig. 67.3 a

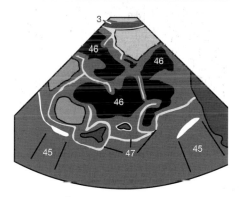

Fig. 67.3 b

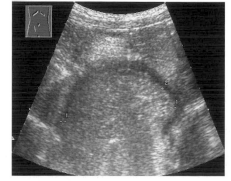

Fig. 67.4 a

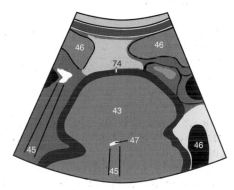

Fig. 67.4 b

Coprostasis

Normally, only the wall of the colon near the transducer can be evaluated, because the colon contains so much air that it usually precludes any visualization of the lumen or opposite wall. Especially in older patients, however, fecal retention can occur (coprostasis, **Fig. 68.1**), shown here in the transverse colon **(43)** without gas, which allows good evaluation of both walls of the colon.

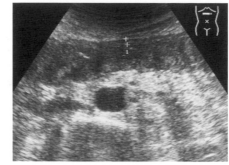

Fig. 68.1 a

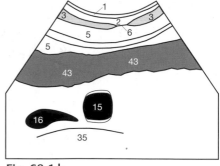

Fig. 68.1 b

Colitis

In inflammatory thickening of the colon wall **(74)** as manifestation of colitis, the haustral indentations can become much more prominent than usual, as seen here in the sigmoid colon **(Fig. 68.2)**. Alternatively, mural thickening of the colon can be ischemic, as seen in mesenteric infarction or venous thrombosis.

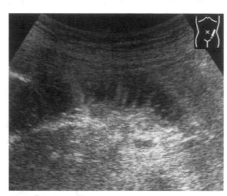

Fig. 68.2 a

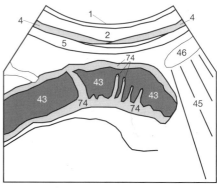

Fig. 68.2 b

Diverticulitis

A possible complication of colon diverticula is a localized diverticulitis. **Figure 68.3** delineates the diverticular neck **(∗)** between the normal lumen **(43)** and the hypoechoic diverticulum **(54)**. Take note of the thickened colon wall **(74)**, which is also seen on the CT performed on this patient **(Fig. 68.4)**. The rectosigmoid junction **(43)** is still well demarcated from the hypodense fatty tissue, while the fatty tissue immediately next to the diverticulum **(54)** is indistinctly demarcated and edematously thickened (white arrow). **Figure 68.5** shows air **(47)** in a small diverticulum with thickening of the adjacent intestinal wall **(74)** as early stage of a diverticulitis.

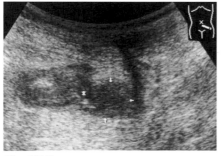

Fig. 68.3 a

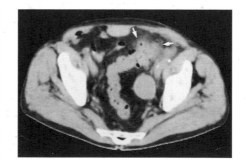

Fig. 68.4 a

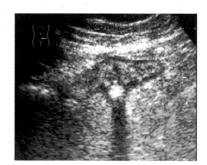

Fig. 68.5 a

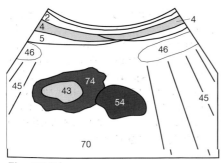

Fig. 68.3 b

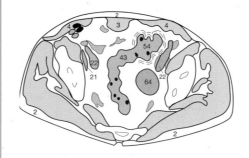

Fig. 68.4 b

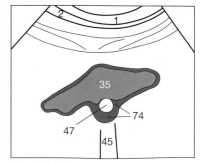

Fig. 68.5 b

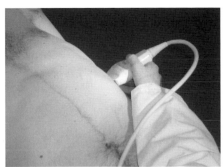

Fig. 69.1

Examination Technique

The spleen is primarily visualized with the patient supine. It is best to ask the patient to slide to the left to make it easier to place the transducer posterolaterally parallel to the intercostal space **(Fig. 69.1)**. The examiner should stand up or sit on the right side of the examination table to have an adequate reach. The examination is done in expiration to exclude the left lung base **(47)** and eliminate any acoustic shadowing **(45)** that may hide the spleen **(37) (Fig. 69.2)**. Even then, the sections of the spleen just beneath the diaphragm **(13)** are often difficult to see. Alternatively, the patient can be examined in the right lateral decubitus position **(Fig. 69.2a)**, but the supine position usually is preferable. The lower pole of the spleen occasionally can be obscured by adjacent intestinal loops **(43)**.

Spleen Size

The normal splenic measurements in adults are 4 cm x 7 cm x 11 cm ("4711" rule), whereby the longitudinal diameter **(L)** can reach 13 cm (instead of 11 cm) without any pathologic implication, for instance after infectious mononucleosis. The maximum diameter **(D**, measured from the hilum to the diaphragmatic capsule of the spleen) has more relevance: If it measures 6 cm (rather than 4 cm), a lymphatic disease should be excluded with additional tests, unless a venous congestion due to portal hypertension is present.

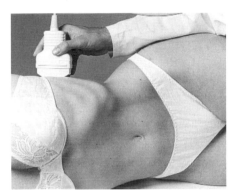

Fig. 69.2 a

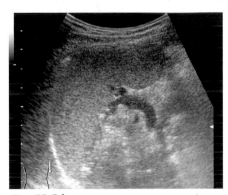

Fig. 69.2 b

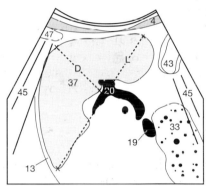

Fig. 69.2 c

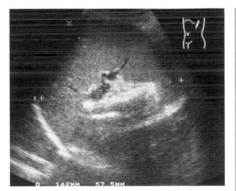

Fig. 69.3 a

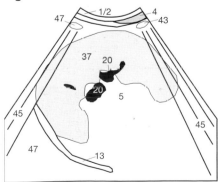

Fig. 69.3 b

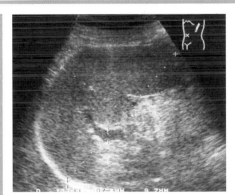

Fig. 69.4 a

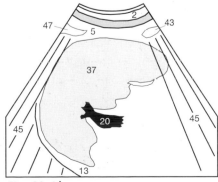

Fig. 69.4 b

Curtain Trick

In some patients, the upper part of the spleen **(37)** is hidden by acoustic shadows **(45)**, either spontaneously or after deep inspiration, with the lung **(47)** extending too far into the costo-diaphragmatic recess **(Fig. 69.3)**. In this situation, one can take advantage of the slower upward retraction of the spleen relative to the lung during slow but still swift expiration following maximal inspiration.

This relative motion makes the acoustic shadow recede like a "curtain." The examiner has to watch for the right moment and then tell the patient to stop exhaling. This maneuver often succeeds in visualizing the regions of the spleen immediately beneath the diaphragm (along the left border of the image in **Figure 69.4**).

Many conditions are accompanied by a diffuse, homogeneous enlargement of the spleen. The differential diagnosis includes portal hypertension (**Fig. 70.2**), which shows the splenic vein (20) to be dilated and its branches prominent at the splenic hilum. Frequently, a viral infection or a possible remote infection with the Epstein-Barr virus accounts for a splenomegaly. In some cases, healed infectious mononucleosis can leave behind a slight to moderate splenomegaly for life without any clinical significance.

Systemic Hematologic Conditions

Splenomegaly typically accompanies systemic hematologic diseases, such as acute or chronic lymphatic leukemia (CLL). **Figure 70.1** shows a spleen including an adjacent accessory spleen (86) and the tail of the pancreas (33) next to the splenic hilum in a patient with leukemia. In principle, all conditions with an increased turnover of erythrocytes, such as hemolytic anemias or polycythemia, are to be considered. These cases can have a considerably enlarged spleen that might extend into the pelvis (**Fig. 70.3**) and exhibit focal infarcts (**Fig. 71.1**). The "kissing phenomenon" may be observed, which refers to a massive splenomegaly with the spleen displacing the stomach and touching the left hepatic lobe.

When evaluating the spleen, it is important to look for evidence of any rotundness. The original crescentic configuration with its pointed poles gets lost, and the poles become rounded or blunted (**Fig. 70.1**). Ectopic splenic tissue, which occasionally occurs as an embryologic remnant in the splenic bed, can also undergo hypertrophy if stimulated. Consequently, visible accessory spleens (86) at the hilum (**Fig. 70.1**) or lower splenic pole do not infrequently accompany a diffuse splenomegaly. They have the same echogenicity as the remaining splenic parenchyma (37) and are sharply demarcated. Their differentiation from enlarged lymph nodes (55), however, may pose a problem, as illustrated in **Figure 70.3**.

Suggestion

Neither size nor echogenicity of the enlarged spleen reveals the nature of the underlying disease. If the sonographic examination of the abdomen unexpectedly detects a splenomegaly, all accessible nodal bearing areas of the abdomen (para-aortal, at the porta hepatis, para-iliac and cervical) should be scrutinized for lymphadenopathy as presumptive evidence of a systemic hematologic condition. Furthermore, portal hypertension should be excluded by measuring the luminal diameter of the splenic vein (normal value < 10 mm), portal vein (normal value < 15 mm) and superior mesenteric vein, and by searching for portocaval collaterals at the porta hepatis.

The documentation of the spleen size should be as accurate as possible in order for follow-up examinations to determine whether the spleen has regressed or progressed, e.g., after a resolved viral infection or a course of chemotherapy in the interim, depending on the underlying disease. Keep this in mind when you perform the initial examination.

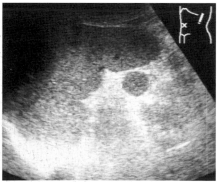

Fig. 70.1 a

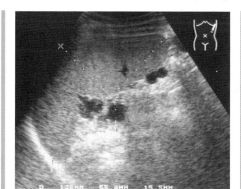

Fig. 70.2 a

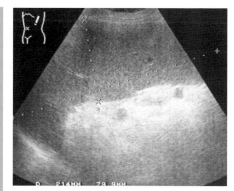

Fig. 70.3 a

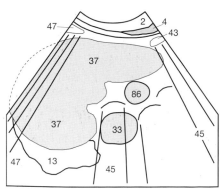

Fig. 70.1 b

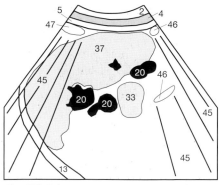

Fig. 70.2 b

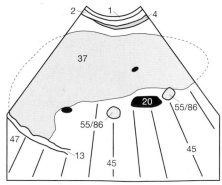

Fig. 70.3 b

Splenic Infarcts

A rapidly progressive splenomegaly is especially prone to focal infarcts (71), which in their early stage appear as hypoechoic areas within still-perfused hyperechoic areas (Fig. 71.1). Supplemental color-coded duplex sonography can establish the status of the splenic perfusion quickly and non-invasively.

Lymphomatous Infiltration

Non-Hodgkin lymphoma can present with singular or multiple diffusely distributed hypoechoic splenic lesions. An enlarged spleen that still appears homogeneous under strictly conventional sonography can nevertheless harbor lymphomatous foci. The detection rate has markedly increased with the introduction of echo-enhancing contrast media used in combination with harmonic imaging (see page12).

Splenic Hematomas

The definitive exclusion of splenic hematomas is of utmost importance in post-traumatic patients, since a fresh hemorrhage may initially be confined to the parenchyma or subcapsular space. Only after some delay (in about 50% of cases within the first week), the splenic capsule can rupture, bringing on a life-threatening hemorrhage into the abdominal cavity (delayed splenic rupture). Carefully scrutinize the splenic parenchyma for hypoechoic areas and the splenic capsule for delicate hypoechoic double contours to exclude such a process. Some splenic hematomas (50) are heterogeneous (Fig. 71.2) or isoechoic with the surrounding splenic parenchyma (37). The arrow (←) in Figure 71.2 points to the site where you have to search for (anechoic) free intra-abdominal fluid (as evidence of hemorrhage) in the supine patient. It is located along the abdominal aspect of the diaphragm (13), posterior to the upper polar spleen.

Hyperechoic Lesions

Spherical and homogeneous hyperechoic lesions that are sharply demarcated from the splenic parenchyma generally represent benign splenic hemangiomas, which have features identical to those of hepatic hematomas (Fig. 37.2). Alternative considerations are hyperechoic calcific lesions following an infection with tuberculosis or histoplasmosis, or accompanying cirrhosis. Multiple echogenic foci (53) make the spleen appear like a "starry sky" (Fig. 71.3) and also present post-infectious scars. Splenic abscesses and the rarely occurring splenic metastases can have a rather varied sonographic morphology, depending on duration and state of the immune system. Simple, reliable differential diagnostic criteria do not exist.

Splenic Cysts

Congenital splenic cysts are anechoic and less common than hepatic cysts. Sonographically, they do not differ from hepatic cysts (see page 37). Acquired splenic cysts develop after trauma or infarcts, or as part of a parasitic infestation. Figure 71.4 shows a CT with cysts containing clearly radiating septations (➘) as manifestation of echinococcosis involving the liver and spleen.

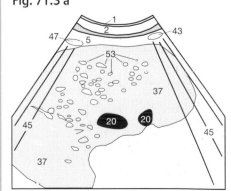

Fig. 71.4

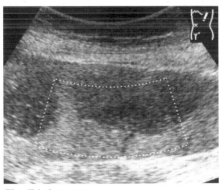

Fig. 71.1 a

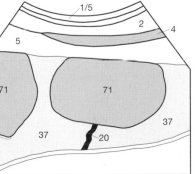

Fig. 71.1 b

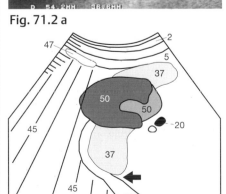

Fig. 71.2 a

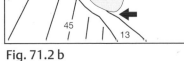

Fig. 71.2 b

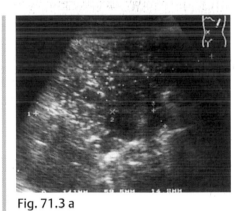

Fig. 71.3 a

Fig. 71.3 b

Splenic Size in Pediatrics

While the "4711 rule" applies with the afore-mentioned restrictions to adults, the size of the spleen in children is measured cranio-caudally along the median axillary line (not parallel to the intercostal space), and is stated relative to the body length (according to Weitzel D.: Sonographic Organometrics in Childhood, Mainz)

Body length[cm]	Length of the spleen [cm]		
	M – 2 SD	$\overline{m}$	M – 2 SD
Newborns	2.90	4.07	5.24
< 55	2.13	2.91	3.69
55 – 70	2.44	3.46	4.48
71 – 85	2.23	3.71	5.19
86 – 100	2.61	4.69	6.77
101 – 110	3.02	4.88	6.74
111 – 120	3.38	5.26	7.14
121 – 130	3.37	5.31	6.87
131 – 140	4.10	5.96	7.82
141 – 150	4.61	5.81	7.01
>150	4.36	6.18	8.00

Spleen: Quiz for Self-Assessment

In our workshops for students and physicians, the sonographic evaluation of the spleen has again and again presented a unique challenge. It is of interest that more than 90% of all participants place the transducer along the anterior (instead of the posterior) axillary line and run into difficulties with acoustic shadowing of the colon or small intestine. Therefore, practice the correct visualization with your fellow student and keep in mind the necessity of standing up to extend your reach. Here are the other learning goals. The answers to quiz questions 1 to 4 are found on the preceding pages, and the answer to the image quiz is at the end of the book on page 108.

1. Write down the normal size measurements of the spleen in adults, and put a splenomegaly in perspective.

2. What trick do you know to visualize the subdiaphragmatic aspect of the spleen when you encounter superimposed pulmonary air? How does it work?

3. Imagine you have a patient with multiple injuries, who has or could have sustained a blunt abdominal trauma. What do you look for sonographically, and where do you place the transducer for that purpose?

4. You discover a splenomegaly unexpectedly. How do you proceed?

5. Systematically evaluate the adjacent image. Approach it sequentially, as recommended in the primer on sonography on page 110, to channel your thoughts into a meaningful direction.

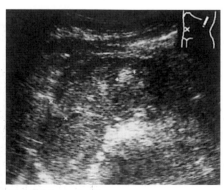

Fig. 72.1

Prostate Gland

Transabdominal sonography of the reproductive organs requires a distended urinary bladder (38) to avoid interfering acoustic shadows (45) by displacing the air-containing intestinal loops (46) superiorly and laterally. The prostate gland (42) is at the bladder floor anterior to the rectum (43) and is seen on suprapubic transverse and sagittal sections (Fig. 73.1).

Prostatic Hypertrophy

The normal prostate gland should not measure more than 5 cm x 3 cm x 3 cm and its calculated volume should not exceed 25 ml (A x B x C x 0.5). A high percentage of older men have prostatic hypertrophy (Fig. 73.2), which can cause voiding difficulties and lead to increased bladder trabeculation (Fig. 58.2). An enlarged prostate gland (42) elevates and indents the floor of the bladder (38), with the bladder wall (77) usually delineated as a smooth, hyperechoic line (Fig. 73.2).

Prostate cancer (54) generally arises in the peripheral zone of the gland. It can invade the bladder wall and eventually protrude into the bladder lumen (Fig. 73.3). Increasing urethral compression can lead to hypertrophy of the musculature of the bladder wall (77), which becomes thickened sonographically (Fig. 73.3).

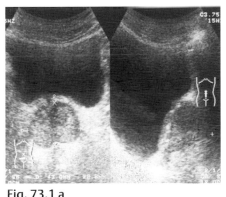

Fig. 73.1 a

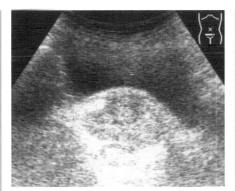

Fig. 73.2 a

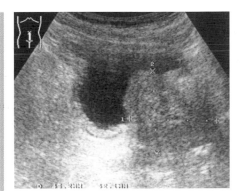

Fig. 73.3 a

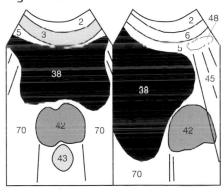

Fig. 73.1 b

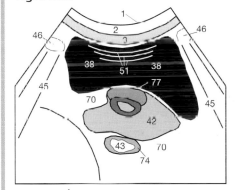

Fig. 73.2 b

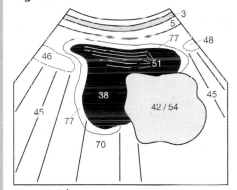

Fig. 73.3 b

Testes and Scrotum

The adult testis (98) is normally homogeneously hypoechoic and clearly demarcated from the scrotal layers (100). It measures about 3 cm x 4 cm on the longitudinal section (Fig. 73.4). The upper testicular pole is capped with the epididymis (99), which extends along the testicular surface. In children, an undescended testis should be excluded on the cross-sectional image (see page 74), which must show both testes next to each other in the scrotum.

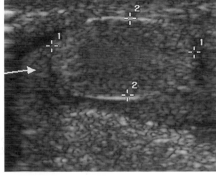

Fig. 73.4 a

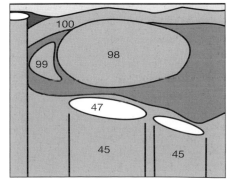

Fig. 73.4 b

Undescended Testis

If both testes are not in the scrotum at 3 months, the localization of an undescended or ectopic testis has to be addressed. The testis (**98**) is frequently found in the inguinal canal near the abdominal wall (**2/5**) as shown in **Figure 74.1**. If sonography fails to localize the undescended testis, MRI should be employed for further evaluation. Because of its risk for malignant degeneration, it is important to find an undescended or ectopic testis.

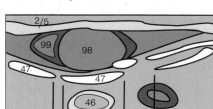

Fig. 74.1 a

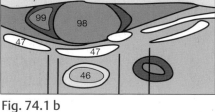

Fig. 74.1 b

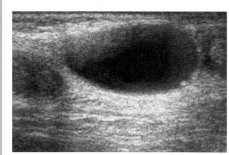

Fig. 74.2

Orchitis / Epididymitis

The differential diagnosis of sudden-onset severe scrotal pain that radiates into the inguinal region must consider a testicular or epididymal infection, in addition to an incarcerated hernia. Testicular tissue can tolerate an ischemia for only about 6 hours before irreversible necrosis sets in. In case of an infection, Doppler sonography shows perfusion with arterial pulses in the flow profile (↘ in **Fig. 74.2**), with the affected side frequently even showing hyperperfusion. Torsion leads to a considerably reduced or absent testicular perfusion in comparison with the contralateral testis.

Orchitis or epididymitis typically shows an edematous enlargement of the testis (**98**) or epididymis (**99**) as well as a multilayered thickening of the scrotal layers (**100**), as shown in **Figure 74.3**. Equivocal findings can be resolved by contralateral comparison.

Hydrocele / Inguinal Hernia

A homogeneous anechoic fluid accumulation (**Fig. 74.4**) is either a hydrocele (**64**) or a varicocele. A varicocele enlarges with the Valsalva maneuver and shows flow on color duplex sonography. Occasionally, herniated bowel (**46**) is seen in the inguinal canal or scrotum together with a hydrocele (**64**) next to the normal testis (**98**, **Fig. 74.5**).

Malignant testicular tumors usually present as heterogeneous changes in the testicular parenchyma. Malignant but still well-differentiated seminomas can be homogeneous with mostly unremarkable sonographic morphology.

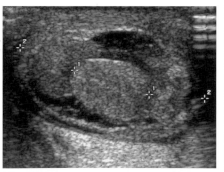

Fig. 74.3 a

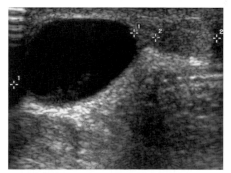

Fig. 74.4 a

Fig. 74.5 a

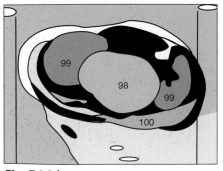

Fig. 74.3 b

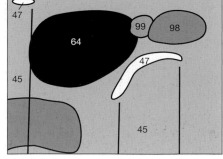

Fig. 74.4 b

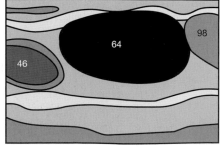

Fig. 74.5 b

The transabdominal visualization (**Fig. 75.1**) of the uterus (**39**) including ovaries (**91**), vagina (**41**) and rectum (**43**) requires a distended urinary bladder as acoustic window. Because of the necessary penetration, low frequencies around 3.5 MHz are used, with corresponding limited resolution. Endosonography offers an alternative with higher spatial resolution (see below).

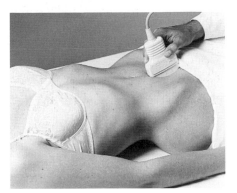

Fig. 75.1 a

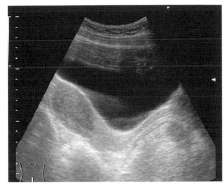

Fig. 75.1 b

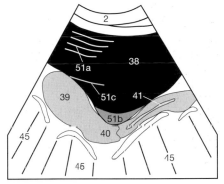

Fig. 75.1 c

Endovaginal Sonography

Because of the proximity to the target organs, transvaginal transducers (**Fig. 75.2**) can be operated at a higher frequency (5 to 10 MHz) with corresponding higher spatial resolution (see page 9). Endosonography has the additional advantage that the urinary bladder need not be full. An assortment of electronic and mechanical transducers with variable imaging sectors (70 to 180 degrees) is available. Transducers with an eccentric sound beam must be turned 180 degrees to visualize the contralateral ovary.

In comparison to transabdominal imaging, the visualization from below causes the endovaginal images to display the findings "upside down." The sound waves propagate from the bottom to the top of the image (**Fig. 75.3**). This orientation shows the

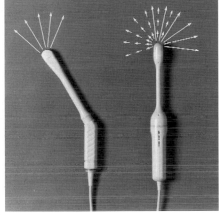

Fig. 75.2 a

intestinal loops with acoustic shadows (**45**) in the upper half of the image, and the uterus (**39**) and cervical region (**40**) in the lower half, near the transducer.

Image Orientation

The sagittal plane is preferably displayed as if the patient is seen from the left.

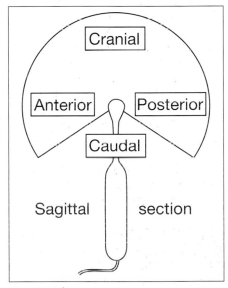

Fig. 75.2 b

The urinary bladder (**38**) and other anterior body structures are on the left side of the image (**Fig. 75.3**), and the cervix (**40**) and other posterior structures are on the right side.

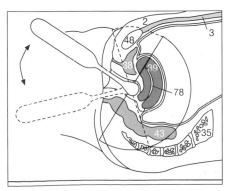

Fig. 75.3 a

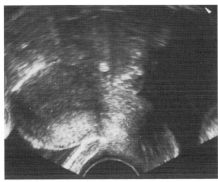

Fig. 75.3 b

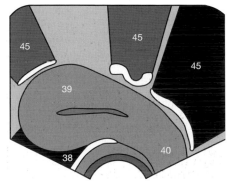

Fig. 75.3 c

The width of the endometrium **(78)** varies with the menstrual cycle. Immediately after menstruation, only a thin, hyperechoic, central line is observed **(Fig. 76.1)**. Around the time of ovulation, the endometrium **(78)** is demarcated (✎) from the myometrium **(39)** by a thin hyperechoic rim **(Fig. 76.2)**.

After the ovulation, the secretory endometrium increasingly loses its central echo (➡ in **Fig. 76.3**) until the endometrium becomes hyperechoic throughout.

The normally homogeneous, hyperechoic myometrium can be traversed by vessels, which appear as anechoic areas.

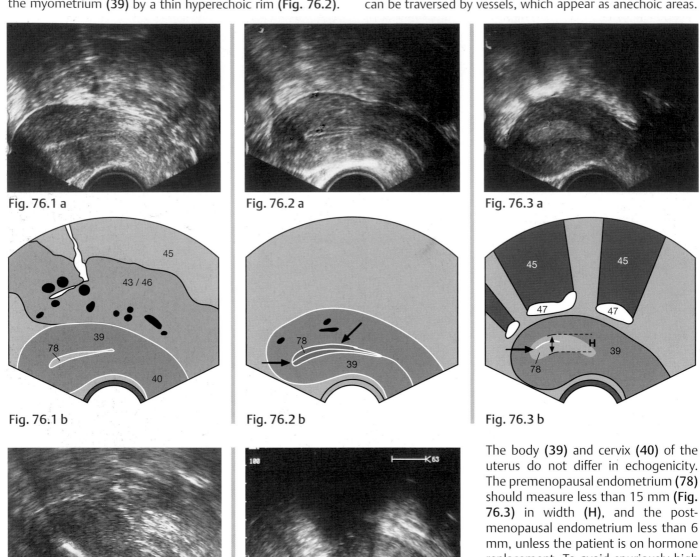

Fig. 76.1 a

Fig. 76.2 a

Fig. 76.3 a

Fig. 76.1 b

Fig. 76.2 b

Fig. 76.3 b

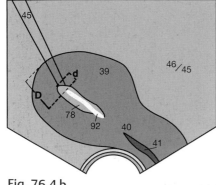

Fig. 76.4 a

Fig. 76.4 b

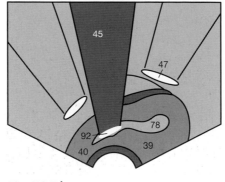

Fig. 76.5 a

Fig. 76.5 b

The body **(39)** and cervix **(40)** of the uterus do not differ in echogenicity. The premenopausal endometrium **(78)** should measure less than 15 mm **(Fig. 76.3)** in width **(H)**, and the postmenopausal endometrium less than 6 mm, unless the patient is on hormone replacement. To avoid spuriously high values due to oblique sectioning, the measurements should be exclusively obtained on longitudinal uterine sections.

Intrauterine Devices (IUD)

An IUD **(92)** is easily recognized by its high echogenicity with acoustic shadowing **(45)** and should be located at the fundus in the uterine cavity. The distance between the IUD **(d)** and the fundal extension of the endometrium should be less than 5 mm, and to the outer surface of the fundus **(D)** less than 20 mm **(Fig. 76.4)**. Wider distances **(Fig. 76.5)** suggest a displaced IUD close to the cervix **(40)** with a less reliable contraceptive effect.

The normal uterus is covered with a hyperechoic serosa and shows a homogeneous hypoechoic myometrium **(39)**. Myomas (fibroids) **(54)** are the most common benign uterine tumors. They arise from the smooth musculature and usually occur in the uterine body. For surgical planning of a myomectomy, myomas are categorized as intra-/transmural **(Fig. 77.1)**, submucosal **(Fig. 77.2)**, and subserosal projecting from the outer uterine surface **(Fig. 77.3)**. A submucosal myoma can easily be mistaken for an endometrial polyp **(65)** **(Fig. 77.2)**.

Myomas have a homogeneous or concentrically laminated echo pattern with sharp demarcation and a smooth surface. They can contain calcifications with acoustic shadowing or central necroses. The size of myomas should be accurately measured and documented to exclude rapid progression on serial examination as evidence of a rare sarcomatous degeneration. In early pregnancy, a sudden enlargement of a myoma can be benign in nature.

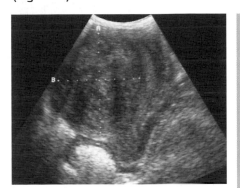

Fig. 77.1 a

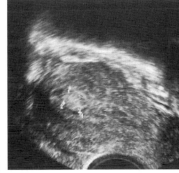

Fig. 77.2 a

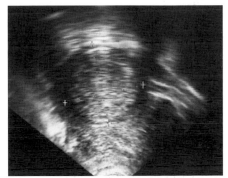

Fig. 77.3 a

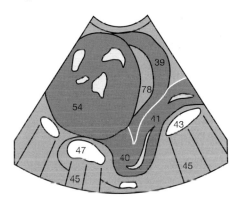

Fig. 77.1 b

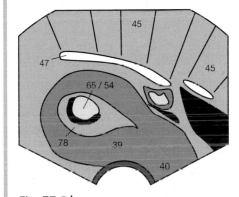

Fig. 77.2 b

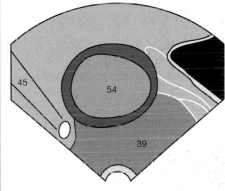

Fig. 77.3 b

Postmenopausal administration of estrogens can induce endometrial hyperplasia **(Fig. 77.4)** through estrogen-secreting ovarian tumors or persistent follicles, with persistent high estrogen levels creating the risk for degeneration of the endometrial hyperplasia into an adenocarcinoma **(54) (Fig. 77.6)**. Malignant criteria are an endometrium that measures more than 6 mm after and 15 mm before menopause, exhibits a heterogeneous echo pattern and is irregularly demarcated, as seen in **Figure 77.6**.

A hypoechoic collection of blood ( ) in the uterine cavity (hematometra) can be caused by postinflammatory adhesions in the cervical canal following conization or by a cervix tumor **(Fig. 77.5)**.

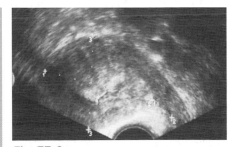

Fig. 77.6 a

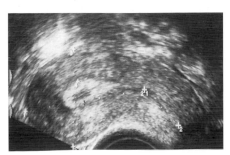

Fig. 77.4

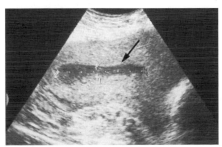

Fig. 77.5

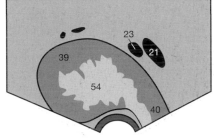

Fig. 77.6 b

Volumetry

The ovaries (91) are visualized on a superolaterally oriented sagittal section (Fig. 78.1) and are usually located in the immediate vicinity of the iliac vessels (23). The transverse diameter is added for measuring the ovarian volume. The product of the three axis diameters multiplied by 0.5 is an adequate estimate of the ovarian volume. In women, the values range from 5.5 to 10 cm³, with a mean of 8 cm³. The ovarian volume is not affected by preceding pregnancies, but continuously decreases postmenopausally from about 3.5 to 2.5 cm³, depending on the number of years since menopause.

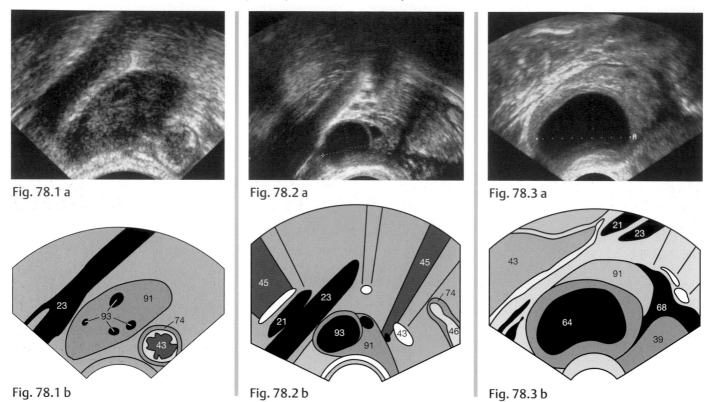

Fig. 78.1 a

Fig. 78.2 a

Fig. 78.3 a

Fig. 78.1 b

Fig. 78.2 b

Fig. 78.3 b

Cycle Phases

In the first days of a new cycle, several follicles (93) are normally visible and appear as 4 mm to 6 mm small anechoic cysts within the ovary. Beginning with the 10th day of the cycle (Fig. 78.2), a dominant follicle appears that measures about 10 mm in diameter (Graafian follicle). It shows linear growth of about 2 mm/day to reach a pre-ovulation diameter of 1.8 mm to 2.5 mm. The remaining follicles shrink in the meantime.

For infertility treatment and in vitro fertilization (IVF), tight sonographic monitoring can trace the follicular maturation and even occasionally determine the time of ovulation endosonographically. Signs of imminent ovulation are a follicle size exceeding 2 cm, a small wall-based cumulus oophoron, and a crenulated follicular wall. Following the ovulation, the Graafian follicle disappears or at least markedly decreases in size. At the same time, free fluid may become detectable in the cul-de-sac.

Invading vessels transform the ruptured follicle into the progesterone-producing corpus luteum, which remains visible for only a few days as a hyperechoic area at the site of the former follicle. In case of conception, the corpus luteum persists and can remain visible as a corpus luteum cyst (64) up to the 14th gestational week (Fig. 78.3).

Abnormal folliculogenesis includes premature follicular luteinization with missed ovulation and formation of a follicular cyst (64 in Fig. 78.4). It should always be kept in mind that a follicular cyst larger than 3 mm for more than one menstrual cycle may represent a persistent follicle (see next page).

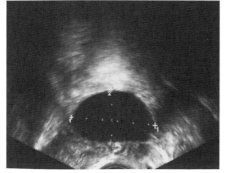

Fig. 78.4 a

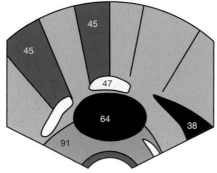

Fig. 78.4 b

An ovarian cyst exceeding 5 cm in diameter (see page 78) is suspicious for tumor. In particular, malignancy must be considered for a cyst with septa and/or solid internal echoes (↖) or increased wall thickness (Fig. 79.1). Similar features are found in dermoid cysts (Fig. 79.2), which comprise 15% of unilateral ovarian tumors. Their internal echoes (↘) correspond to fat, hair and other tissues. They are mostly benign and only rarely become malignant.

These findings must be separated from hemorrhagic or endometriotic cysts, which either contain intraluminal fluid levels (→) (Fig. 79.3) or are completely filled with homogeneous blood products (50) (Fig. 79.4). Do you know why the fluid level in **Figure 79.3** is almost vertically oriented? The answer is found on page 109.

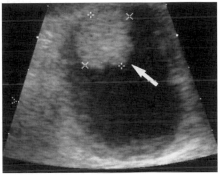

Fig. 79.1

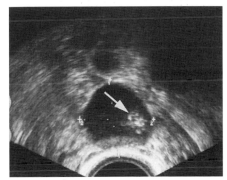

Fig. 79.2

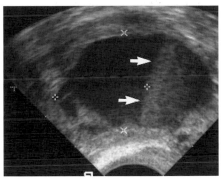

Fig. 79.3

Infertility Therapy

Measuring the hormone levels of an externally stimulated cycle does not allow a definitive exclusion of hyperstimulated ovaries (Fig. 79.5) or a reliable statement about the number of stimulated follicles (93). Sonographic tracking of the number of growing Graafian follicles can determine whether the stimulation is appropriate.

About 5% of women have polycystic ovaries (PCO) associated with anovulation, often induced by adrenal hyperandrogenism. The typical features of the PCO syndrome are multiple small cysts (64) that are primarily arranged peripherally around a central stroma (91) of increased echogenicity (Fig. 79.6). Hormone stimulation can treat such ovulatory causes of infertility.

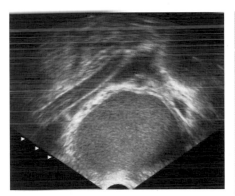

Fig. 79.4 a

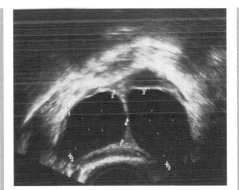

Fig. 79.5 a

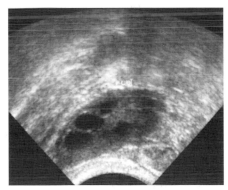

Fig. 79.6 a

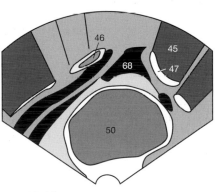

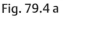

Fig. 79.4 b

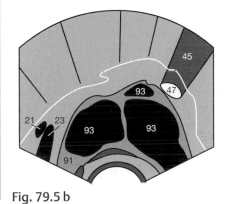

Fig. 79.5 b

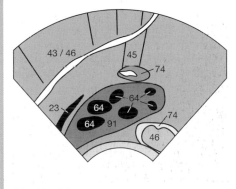

Fig. 79.6 b

Pregnancy testing is not confined to measuring beta-hCG in the maternal blood or urine. Additional sonographic examinations cannot only confirm the pregnancy, but also exclude an ectopic pregnancy (EP). Furthermore, sonography can detect multifetal gestations **(Figs. 81.3/4)**.

The endosonographic threshold for detecting the chorionic cavity of an early intrauterine pregnancy (here is a picture of my first daughter, **Fig. 80.1**) begins at about 2 mm to 3 mm. This size is generally reached 14 days after conception, corre-

sponding to a gestational (menstrual) age of 4 weeks and 3 days.

The small chorionic cavity embedded in the hyperechoic endometrium **(78)** of the uterine cavity **(39)** enlarges at a rate of about 1.1 mm per day to become the gestational sac **(101)**, in which the embryonic disc **(95)** is later identified **(Fig. 80.2)**. Embryonic cardiac activities begin at 6 weeks' gestational age with a heart rate of 80 to 90 beats per minute. Doppler sonography should not be routinely applied to determine the cardiac rate, as long as the embryonic development is proceeding normally (see below).

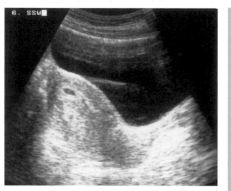

Fig. 80.1 a

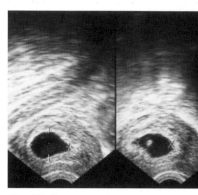

Fig. 80.2 a

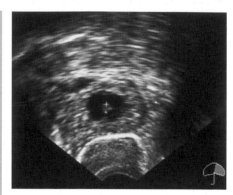

Fig. 80.3 a

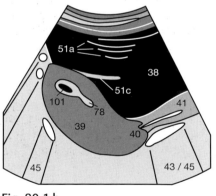

Fig. 80.1 b

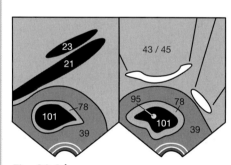

Fig. 80.2 b

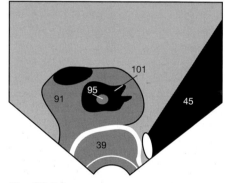

Fig. 80.3 b

If an embryo is not identified in the chorionic cavity when expected, the gestational age should be checked first. If a follow-up examination shows growth retardation of a still empty chorionic cavity (see page 82), a blighted ovum or anembryonic pregnancy is present, which occurs in about 5% of all gestations.

Ectopic Pregnancy (EP)

In an ectopic pregnancy **(Fig. 80.3)**, the gestational sac **(95)** is outside the uterus **(39)**. Because of its severe consequences, it should not be missed.

Safety of Diagnostic Ultrasound in Fetal Screening

According to the guidelines of the American Institute of

Ultrasound in Medicine (AIUM), sound energies below 100 mW / cm^2 or 50 J / cm are safe. Since the energies delivered with B-imaging (black / white) are far lower, neither relevant tissue heating nor mutagenic effects can be expected according to current knowledge. This also applies to repeat sonographic examinations during pregnancy. In this context, it should be kept in mind that sound pulses are only emitted during a small fraction of the examination time, with most of the time needed to receive the reflected echoes.

The situation is different for color and pulsed Doppler examinations. For long examination times, these can deliver sound energies that exceed values accepted as safe. Though no evidence of damaging effects of sound waves has been found so far, unnecessary (color) Doppler sonography should be avoided during the sensitive phase of organogenesis in the first trimester. References for these statements are available from the author.

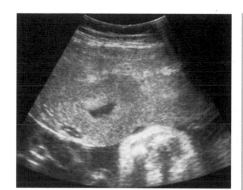

Fig. 81.1 a

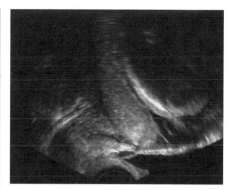

Fig. 81.2 a

The normal location of the placenta is near the fundus along the anterior or posterior uterine wall. In about 20% of cases, the placenta (94) has one or more uni- or multilocular cysts or lacunae (64), which have no functional significance (Fig. 81.1). An association with maternal diabetes or Rhesus incompatibility has been suggested, however.

The definitive location of the placenta cannot be reliably determined before the end of the 2nd trimester, since a placenta previa of an early pregnancy can change to a normal or low-lying placenta (distance to internal os < 5 cm) through increasing stretching of the lower uterine segment.

Three types of a placenta previa are distinguished: complete placenta previa, which totally covers the internal os (40); partial placenta previa, which partially covers the internal os (Fig. 81.2); and marginal placenta previa, which extends to the edge of the internal os. The structural evaluation of the placenta has become less important, since placental and fetal perfusion can be checked with Doppler sonography.

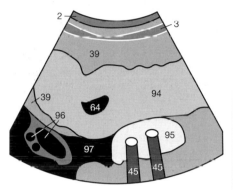

Fig. 81.1 b

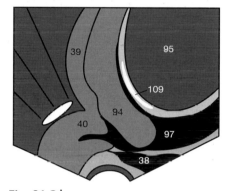

Fig. 81.2 b

Multifetal Gestations

In multifetal gestations, it must be determined whether the gestational sacs (95) share one placenta or are supplied by separate placentas (← in Fig. 81.4). Parents-to-be (and their obstetrician) like to know whether to expect twins (Fig. 81.3) or even triplets (Fig. 81.4). Furthermore, some parents want know whether they should prepare for a daughter (Fig. 81.5) or son (Fig. 81.6).

Gender Determination

Remember to reveal to the parents the gender of the fetus only when asked or it it has been previously requested. Above all, this determination should be accurate. Early in pregnancy, diagnostic errors (?) can occur by mistaking the umbilical cord (↘) for the clitoris or (↖) penis, and by the often indistinguishable appearance of female labia and the male scrotum (→) (Figs. 81.5/6).

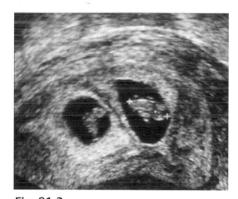

Fig. 81.3

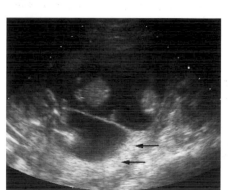

Fig. 81.4

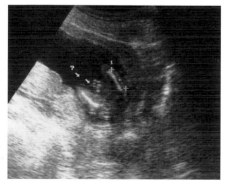

Fig. 81.5

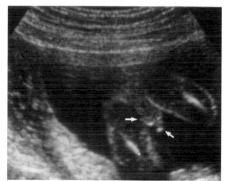

Fig. 81.6

With the help of biometric parameters, sonography can reveal early gestational growth disturbances. Furthermore, sonography can detect fetal malformations. The normal values of the subsequent measurements can be found as tables with median and percentile values (for the German population) on page 119.

Chorionic Cavity Diameter (CD)

The initially anechoic chorionic cavity **(101)** is surrounded by a hyperechoic rim of reactive endometrium **(78)** **(Fig. 82.1)** and becomes visible beginning at the 14th day of the conception. It should be detectable with serum hCG levels above 750 to 1000 U/L – otherwise an ectopic pregnancy must be excluded (see page 80).

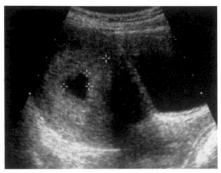

Fig. 82.1 a

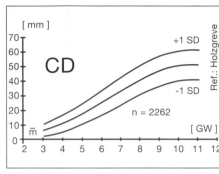

Fig. 82.1 b

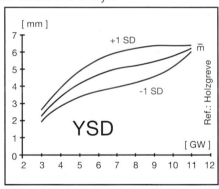

Fig. 82.1 c

Yolk Sac Diameter (YSD)

The yolk sac is a hyperechoic ring structure with an anechoic center that increases to a size of about 5 mm at the 10th gestational week. A yolk sac diameter under 3 mm or above 7 mm implies an increased risk of developmental anomalies.

If the yolk sac is identified within the uterine cavity, an intrauterine pregnancy is established, since the yolk sac is an embryonal structure. **Figure 82.2** shows a yolk sac **(102)** next to the spine **(35)**, belonging to an already older embryo of a gestational age of 7 weeks and 6 days.

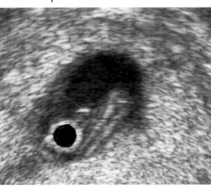

Fig. 82.2 a

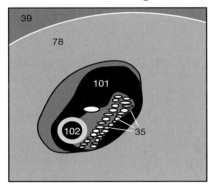

Fig. 82.2 b

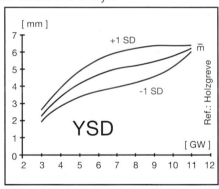

Fig. 82.2 c

Crown Rump Length (CRL)

Beginning at the gestational age of 6 weeks and 3 days, a normal embryo becomes visible and has a measurable crown rump length of 5 mm. At this point in time, the gestational sac measures 15 mm to 18 mm. The crown rump diameter

of a visible embryo **(95)** replaces the chorionic cavity diameter, since it allows a more reliable determination of gestational age (within a few days) up to the 12th gestational week **(Fig. 82.3)**. Thereafter, the biparietal diameter is more accurate (see page 83).

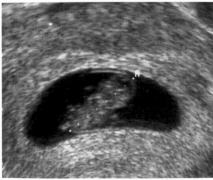

Fig. 82.3 a

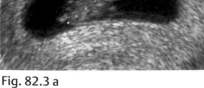

Fig. 82.3 b

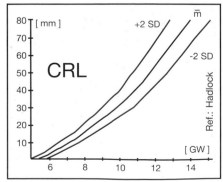

Fig. 82.3 c

Biparietal Diameter (BPD)

Beginning with the 12th gestational week, the biparietal diameter is a more practical and accurate measurement than the crown rump length. The choroid plexus (**104**) appears as a bilateral hyperechoic structure. To obtain exact and reproducible values, the biparietal diameter should be measured on the uninterrupted display of the oval calvarium (**105**) at the same reference level (**Fig. 83.1**). The orientation should be perpendicular to the midline echoes of the falx (**106**), which shows a gap in its frontal third caused by the cavum septi pellucidum. The imaging plane should not include the cerebellum or orbits, since measurements at this level are too far caudal. Biparietal diameter, head circumference (HC) and fronto-occipital diameter (FOD) can be measured at the same reference level. The normal values are found on page 119 and on the pocket-sized cut-out cards.

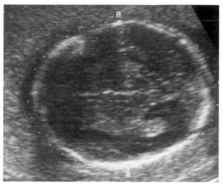

Fig. 83.1 a

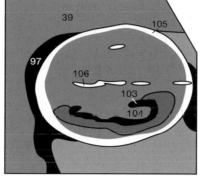

Fig. 83.1 b

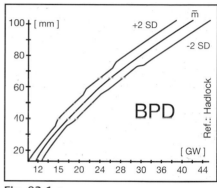

Fig. 83.1 c

Femur Length (FL)

Measuring the ossified femoral diaphysis (**107**) is relatively easy. The long axis of the upper thigh (**108**) should be in transverse position, parallel to the surface axis of the transducer (**Fig. 83.2**). Measurements of other tubular bones are obtained only for clarification when the femoral length falls outside the normal range or serial measurements cross the percentiles, to exclude any growth retardation or any malformations.

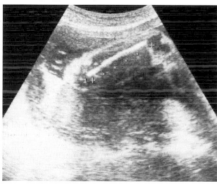

Fig. 83.2 a

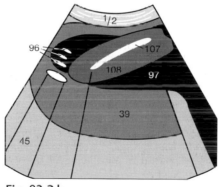

Fig. 83.2 b

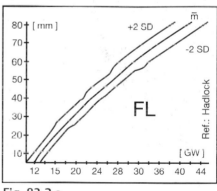

Fig. 83.2 c

Abdominal Circumference (AC)

The abdominal circumference (**Fig. 83.3**) is measured at the level of the liver (**9**), if possible with visualization of the posterior third of the umbilical and portal veins (**11**). The sectioned ribs should appear symmetric to make sure that the abdomen is not sectioned obliquely.

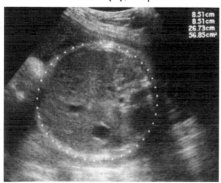

Fig. 83.3 a

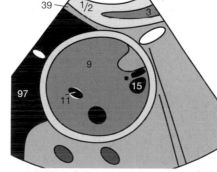

Fig. 83.3 b

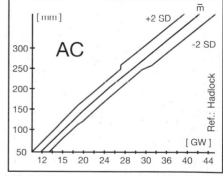

Fig. 83.3 c

Cerebellum

The cerebellum **(110)** is visualized on a transverse section through the posterior cranial fossa **(Fig. 84.1)**. One looks for the physiologic posterior indentation (**←**). Its absence (= "banana sign") indicates a downward displacement of the cerebellum toward the spinal canal **(Fig. 84.2)** as in spina bifida.

For the same reason, the calvarium **(105)** loses its typical oval shape on transverse cerebral sections and resembles a cut lemon (= "lemon sign") with inward scalloping (**↙**) of the frontal bones bilaterally **(Fig. 84.3)**. The echogenic choroid plexus **(104)** is also visualized.

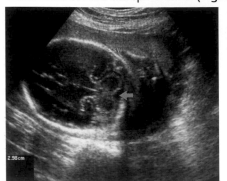

Fig. 84.1 a

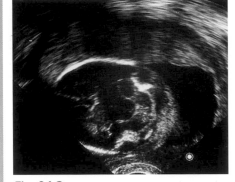

Fig. 84.2 a

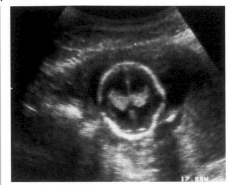

Fig. 84.3 a

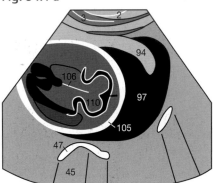

Fig. 84.1 b

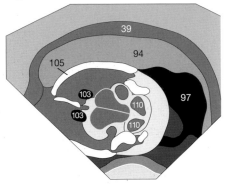

Fig. 84.2 b

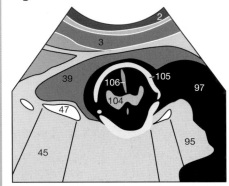

Fig. 84.3 b

CSF Spaces

The choroid plexus can contain small unilateral cysts (**↖**) **(Fig. 84.4)**, which generally lack any clinical significance but have been associated with trisomy 18 and rarely with renal and cardiac malformations. Hydrocephalus **(Fig. 84.5)**, as seen with aqueductal stenosis or spina bifida, is associated with other intra- and extracellular malformations in 70 to 90% of cases.

The reference value for a hydrocephalus is a ventricle-hemisphere ratio exceeding 0.5 after the 20th gestational week. A distinction is made between the ratio of the frontal horn diameter to the hemispheric diameter and of the occipital horn diameter to the hemispheric diameter, which is slightly higher **(Fig. 84.6b)**. Obtaining this measurement can be difficult because the lateral ventricular wall often is not sharply demarcated from the cerebral parenchyma **(Fig. 84.6a)**.

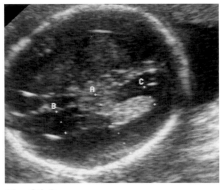

Fig. 84.6 a

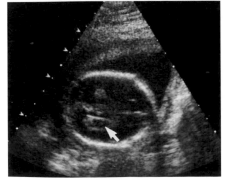

Fig. 84.4

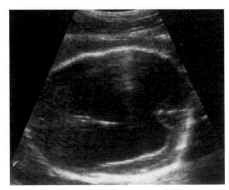

Fig. 84.5

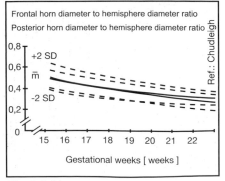

Fig. 84.6 b

Spinal Anatomy

The spine (35) is sagittally scrutinized (Fig. 85.1), coronally visualized (Fig. 85.2), and subsequently scanned cranio-caudally to check for any interruption of the chain formed by the vertebral elements, e.g., spinous processes. It is impor-tant that the transverse sections (Fig. 85.3) show a tight triangle of the three ossification centers (35) for each segment. The fetal aorta (15) is seen anterior to the spine.

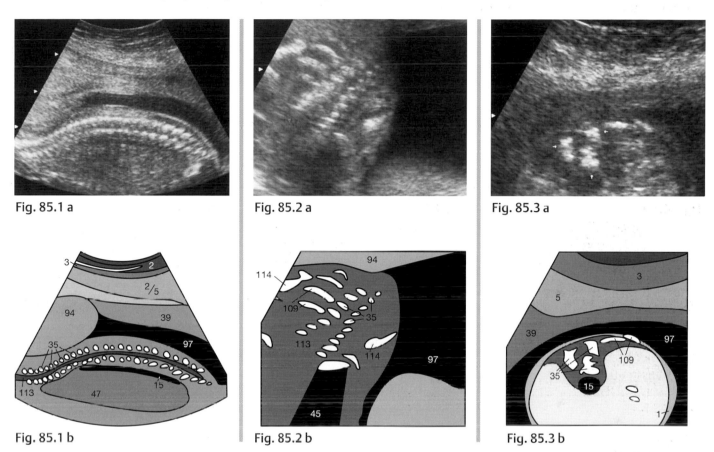

Fig. 85.1 a

Fig. 85.2 a

Fig. 85.3 a

Fig. 85.1 b

Fig. 85.2 b

Fig. 85.3 b

Spina Bifida

Spina bifida is a malformation due to incomplete fusion of the neural tube combined with a variable defect of the vertebral arches. A spina bifida (Fig. 85.4) widens the distance between the posterior ossification centers (✔ ✘). Measuring the maternal serum levels of alpha-feto-protein only allows the diagnosis of an open spina bifida (spina bifida aperta). It does not detect a closed spina bifida (spina bifida occulta).

The fetal cranial findings as indirect cerebral signs of a spina bifida, the so-called "banana" and "lemon" signs, are shown on page 84.

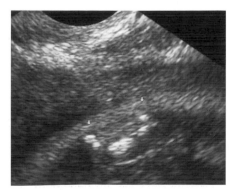

Fig. 85.4 a

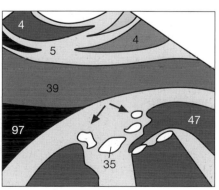

Fig. 85.4 b

Facial Bones

The transverse and coronal sections of the face are generally checked for a decreased (hypotelorism) or increased (hypertelorism) interocular distance, and the sagittal sections for an unusual profile. Clefts of the upper lip and anterior palate are usually laterally located and are best recognized on the coronal plane as an interrupted hyperechoic upper lip, which normally (➡, ↘) is visualized as a continuous structure (**Fig. 86.1**).

Nuchal Translucency

Edema of the cervical subcutaneous layer (nuchal translucency) exceeding 3 mm in width suggests impaired lymphatic drainage if found between the 10th and 14th gestational week (corresponding to a crown rump length between 38 and 84 mm). One-third of these cases are associated with chromosomal abnormalities, such as monosomy X (Turner syndrome), trisomy 21 (Down syndrome) and trisomy 18. To distinguish the nuchal skin from amnion along the fetal skin, it is important to wait for spontaneous fetal activity. Furthermore, a tangentially sectioned nuchal skin can mimic a double contour (↓) (**Fig. 86.2**), which invariably measures less than 3 mm. The risk of a chromosomal abnormality increases with the width of the nuchal translucency and maternal age (**Fig. 86.2c**).

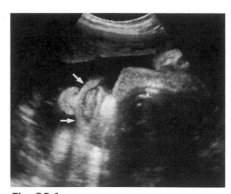

Fig. 86.1

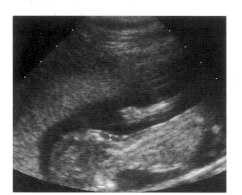

Fig. 86.2 a

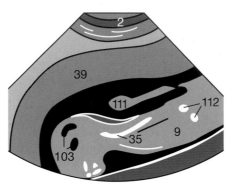

Fig. 86.2 b

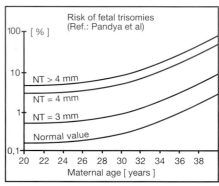

Fig. 86.2 c

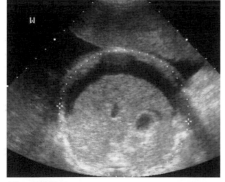

Fig. 86.3 a

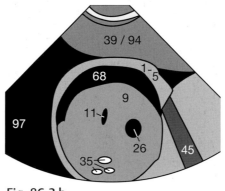

Fig. 86.3 b

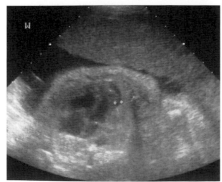

Fig. 86.4 a

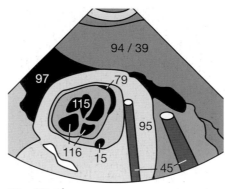

Fig. 86.4 b

Hydrops Fetalis

Increased accumulation of fluid in serous cavities and in the placenta can have several causes, including congestive heart failure, anemia due to infection, congenital fetal anemia, Rhesus incompatibility, chromosomal abnormalities and metabolic disorders.

In monochorionic twins, the hydrops fetalis of one twin is caused by twin-to-twin transfusion through arteriovenous shunts. Aside from ascites (**68** in **Fig. 86.3**) and pleural and pericardial effusion (**79** in **Fig. 86.4**), sonography might show generalized soft-tissue edema.

Checklist for Hydrops Fetalis

- Ascites
- Pleural effusions
- Pericardial effusions
- Generalized soft-tissue edema

The cardiovascular system is the first functioning system of the embryo. From the 6th gestational week on, cardiac contractions are visible. Absent cardiac contractions and arrested growth of the gestational sac, which at this point has often become indistinctly demarcated, speak for a missed abortion, often requiring a D and C.

Doppler and color-coded Doppler sonography should be avoided because of their high sound intensities (see page 80). They should only be applied in suspected growth retardation or cardiac malformation.

Cardiac Anatomy

First, the heart has to be located. At the level of the four-chamber view, one-third of the heart lies to the right of an imaginary line from the spine to the anterior thoracic wall, and two-thirds are to the left of this line. The sagittal section (**Fig. 87.1**) should be oriented to dissect aortic arch (**15**) and origins of the supra-aortic branches, which include the brachiocephalic artery (**117**), the left common carotid artery (**82**) and the left subclavian artery (**123**). Besides visualizing

the valves, the four-chamber view (**Fig. 87.2**) must also display the atria (**116**) and ventricles (**115**), and should exclude ventricular and atrial defects.

By gently tilting the transducer, the inflow tract of the mitral valve (**118**) and the outflow tract of the left ventricle over the aortic valve (**119**) come into view on the so-called "five-chamber view" (**Fig. 87.3**).

Diagnosis of Congenital Cardiac Shunts

A membranous ventricular septal defect is best seen on the five-chamber view. However, definitive exclusion of small atrioventricular defects or cardiovascular shunts requires the additional color-coded echocardiography performed by an experienced examiner.

Even transposition of the great vessels (TGA) can be overlooked on the four-chamber view. It is therefore essential to check not only the crossing of the outflow tracts, but also the aortic and pulmonary valves on the short axis view.

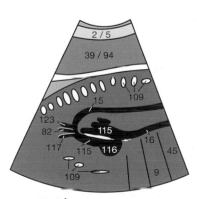

Fig. 87.1 a

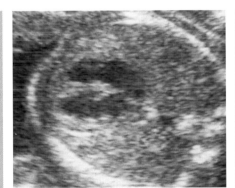

Fig. 87.2 a

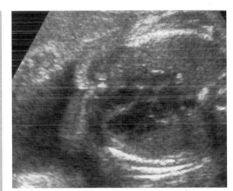

Fig. 87.3 a

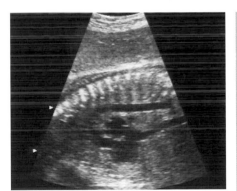

Fig. 87.1 b

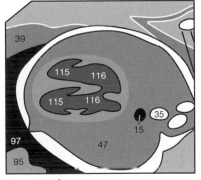

Fig. 87.2 b

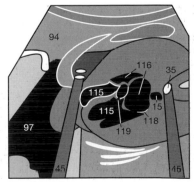

Fig. 87.3 b

GI Tract

Among other signs, the examiner must look for the "double bubble" sign, which suggests a duodenal atresia or stenosis, when evaluating the GI tract. Two adjacent bubbles, which are filled with fluid and consequently anechoic, can represent the stomach and duodenal segment proximal to the obstruction.

The finding should be identified in two planes to avoid a false-positive diagnosis mimicked by a tangentially visualized stomach that is sectioned by the sound beam twice.

Umbilical Hernia and Omphalocele

It should be kept in mind that herniation of fetal bowel **(120)** in the anterior abdominal wall **(Fig. 88.1)** next to the umbilical vessels **(96)** is physiologic until the 11th gestational week. This should not be mistaken for a true omphalocele (a pathologic extrusion of abdominal contents).

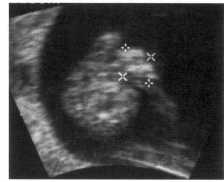

Fig. 88.1 a

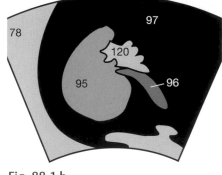

Fig. 88.1 b

Kidneys

Beginning in the 15th gestational week, renal malformations are often indirectly recognized as oligohydramnios, absent amniotic fluid or an empty bladder. At this stage of fetal development, the amniotic fluid represents renal urinary excretion. On the longitudinal section **(Fig. 88.2)** of the normal renal parenchyma **(29)**, the less echogenic medullary pyramids **(30)** and the anechoic pelvis **(31)** can be identified. An overview of the intrauterine growth of the kidneys is shown in **Figure 88.2c**.

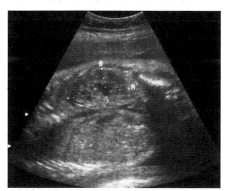

Fig. 88.2 a

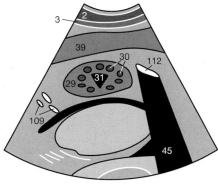

Fig. 88.2 b

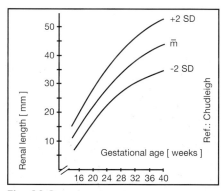

Fig. 88.2 c

Fetal urinary obstruction as caused, for instance, by ureteropelvic junction stenosis, can be best detected on a cross-section of the kidneys **(Fig. 88.3)** by comparing both sides. Cystic renal diseases present either in adulthood (Potter III) or already early as multicystic (Potter II) or microcystic echogenic kidneys (Potter I).

The type Potter III might even be discovered prenatally as diffusely increased renal echogenicity in the presence of a normal amount of amniotic fluid and a full urinary bladder.

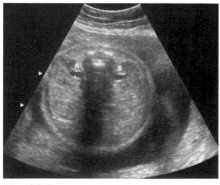

Fig. 88.3 a

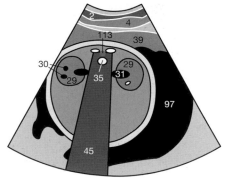

Fig. 88.3 b

Hands

In the 2nd and 3rd trimesters, the hands (**Fig. 89.1**) are checked for completeness of the phalangeal (**121**) and metacarpal (**122**) ossification centers. This cannot only exclude a syndactyly as part of limb-related malformation syndromes, but can also detect polydactylies with supernumerary phalanges (see below).

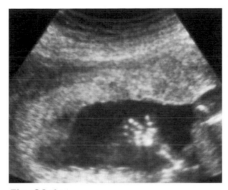

Fig. 89.1 a

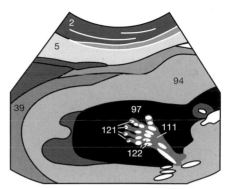

Fig. 89.1 b

Feet

Depending on the intrauterine mobility of the fetus and the experience of the examiner, the feet can be so clearly visualized (**Fig. 89.2**) that metatarsals (**122**) and toes (**121**) can be counted. **Figure 89.3** shows a hexadactyly (6 toes).

Polydactylies are occasionally associated with shortened ribs, a bell-shaped thorax and a consecutive pulmonary hypoplasia.

Clubfoot

Do not forget to rule out a clubfoot (**Fig. 89.4**), which not only encompasses a clubfoot deformity but also positional anomalies and deformed and shortened tubular bones.

A dysplasia of the enchondral ossification as part of achondroplasia is frequently only noticed in the 3rd trimester, showing shortened tubular bones in comparison with the disproportionately large appearing head.

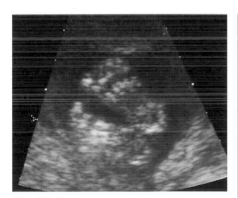

Fig. 89.2 a

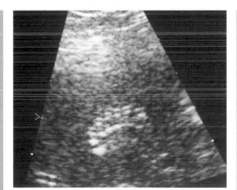

Fig. 89.3 a

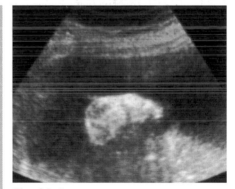

Fig. 89.4 a

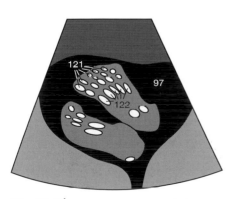

Fig. 89.2 b

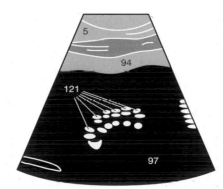

Fig. 89.3 b

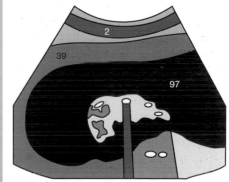

Fig. 89.4 b

In closing of this chapter, you can again test which details you have remembered and in which areas you still must fill knowledge gaps. The answers to quiz questions 1 to 6 can be found on the preceding pages, while the answer to the image question (# 7) is on page 108 at the end of the book.

1. On page 79, you were asked why the fluid level is vertically oriented on the sonographic image of a hemorrhagic endometrial cyst. Do you understand the answer? If not, review the description of the endovaginally obtained sagittal image plane on page 75.

2. An 18-year-old male patient presents with severe pain in the left scrotum, which began about three hours earlier and radiates into the left groin. What is the principal differential diagnosis? How much time do you have to establish the diagnosis? What sonographic methods do you plan to use?

3. How do you recognize sonographically an imminent ovulation? What should change thereafter (after the ovulation)? How many days after the last menstruation or ovulation can conception be sonographically (endovaginally) documented?

4. List six biometric parameters (measurements of fetal organ sizes in prenatal care) next to this text. Next to each, write the gestational weeks for which the respective measurements are meaningful. When is one parameter replaced by another parameter?

5. What are the direct and indirect sonographic criteria of spina bifida? Is testing the mother's serum adequate? Why or why not?

6. What are the renal malformations detectable in the fetus? List at least three sonographic criteria of these malformations.

7. A 58-year-old female patient is sent for a routine gynecologic sonographic examination of the pelvis. The patient had her menopause at age 52 years and has not taken any hormone preparation within the last 5 years. Your endovaginal sonography produces the finding seen in **Figure 90.1**. The endometrium measures 18 mm in cross-sectional width. What is your working diagnosis and how would you proceed?

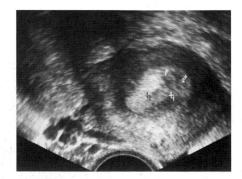

Fig. 90.1

For the examination of newborns and infants, the optimal conditions are not only a quiet environment free of interfering hectic activity, a pre-warmed gel and an infrared light over the examination table, but also the presence of a person close to the child.

The examination is performed through the anterior fontanelle **(135) (Fig. 95.1)** until its closure at the age of about 1 ½ years. With increasing age, the acoustic window gets continuously smaller, making it increasingly more difficult to see the lateral and peripheral cerebral structures, even with maximal tilting of the transducer.

Transducers of proven usefulness are multifrequency sector transducers **(Fig. 91.1c)** with a small contact coupling area and a center frequency of about 3.0 MHz (for infants), 5.0 MHz (from the 6th to 18th month) or 7.5 MHz (for preterm and term newborns). More recently introduced transducers combine the good near-field resolution of linear transducers with a depth dependent diverging beam, to visualize wider cerebral segments **(Fig. 91.1c)**.

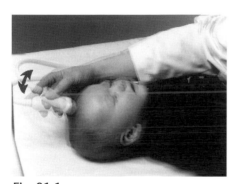

Fig. 91.1 a

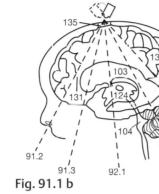

Fig. 91.1 b

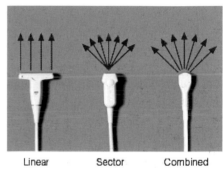

Fig. 91.1 c

The head is scanned in the coronal and sagittal plane (see page 84) with a slow and continuous sweep of the transducer **(Fig. 91.1a, b)**, with passage through and documentation of five standard coronal planes. The most anterior plane

(Fig. 91.2) shows the periventricular white matter **(131)**, which is more hyperechoic than the overlying cortex **(132)**. The transducer sits on the superior sagittal sinus **(136)**.

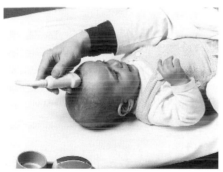

Fig. 91.2 a

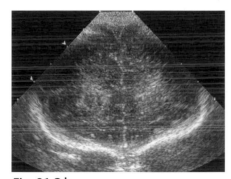

Fig. 91.2 b

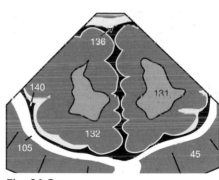

Fig. 91.2 c

The immediately posterior plane **(Fig. 91.3)** intersects the frontal horns of both lateral ventricles **(103)**, which should not contain any hyperechoic choroid plexus at this level. A slight ventricular asymmetry can be physiologic or indicate oblique

sectioning. The shape of the hyperechoic Sylvian fissure **(134)** resembles a 90-degree-rotated Y (compare **Fig. 92.1c**).

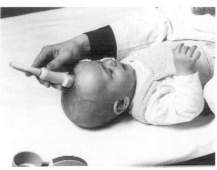

Fig. 91.3 a

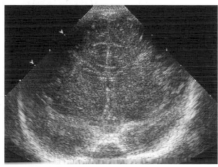

Fig. 91.3 b

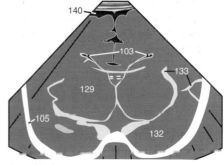

Fig. 91.3 c

The next posterior plane shows the connection between the lateral ventricles (**103**) and the 3rd ventricle (**124**) across the foramen of Monro (**144**) (**Fig. 92.1**). Besides anechoic CSF, the hyperechoic choroid plexus (**104**) is seen in the lumen of the ventricular transition. The hyperechoic choroid plexus should not be mistaken for an equally hyperechoic intraventricular hemorrhage.

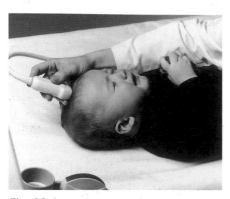

Fig. 92.1 a

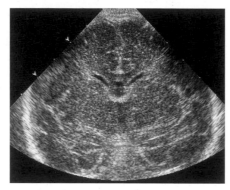

Fig. 92.1 b

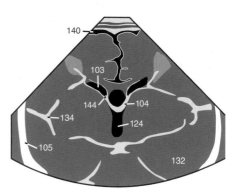

Fig. 92.1 c

With more anterior tilting of the transducer (**Fig. 92.2a**), the sound beam extends further occipitally and visualizes the curved bodies of both lateral ventricles, including the transition to the temporal horns (**Fig. 92.2b**). The width of the lateral ventricles (**103**) and thickness of the choroid plexus (**104**) can be easily determined here. The choroid plexus is normally smoothly outlined. The thalamus, internal capsule and putamen are medially located.

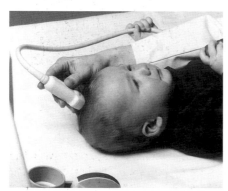

Fig. 92.2 a

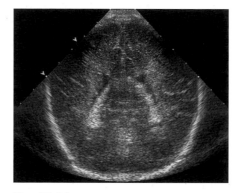

Fig. 92.2 b

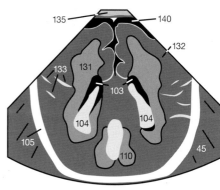

Fig. 92.2 c

Extreme angulation of the transducer (**Fig. 92.3a**) brings into the image the somewhat indistinctly outlined and hyperechoic occipital white matter (**131**) (**Fig. 92.3a**), which surrounds the ventricle in a butterfly-like pattern. Notice the multitude of sulci (**133**) that cross the cortex as hyperechoic lines because of its abundant vascularity and connective tissue. The normal widths of the CSF spaces are demonstrated on the next page.

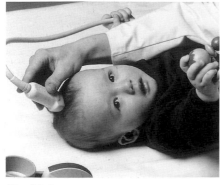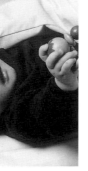

Fig. 92.3 a

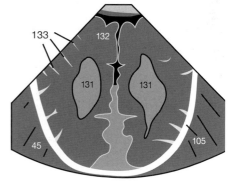

Fig. 92.3 b

Fig. 92.3 c

CSF Spaces

Additional images of the subarachnoid CSF spaces and other superficial structures are obtained with a linear transducer of 5.0 to 7.5 MHz to achieve an adequate resolution (Fig. 93.1). In the neonate, the normal width of the frontal horns (103) measured from the midline complex of the falx (106) to the lateral ventricular wall should not exceed 13 mm. The measurements are made at the level of the foramen of Monro (144) or 3rd ventricle (124). The width of the 3rd ventricle should not exceed 10 mm.

The subarachnoid CSF space is measured at three levels. The interhemispheric fissure (146), measured at he level of two opposite sulci, has a maximal width of 6 mm in the

CSF Spaces in the Newborn		
SCW	Sinocortical width	< 3 mm
CCW	Craniocortical width	< 4 mm
IHW	Interhemispheric width	< 6 mm
LVW	Width of the lateral ventricle, frontal horn	< 13 mm
3rd VW	Width of the 3rd ventricle	< 10 mm

neonate. Sinocortical (147, < 3 mm) and craniocortical (148, < 4 mm) widths are determined to exclude cerebral atrophy (widened subarachnoid CSF space) or an internal hydrocephalus (narrowed subarachnoid CSF space).

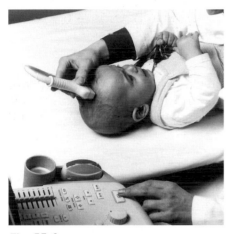

Fig. 93.1 a

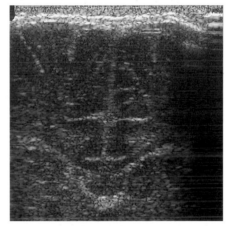

Fig. 93.1 b

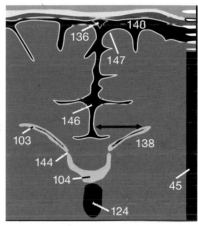

Fig. 93.1 c

Sagittal Plane

After scanning in the coronal plane has been completed, the transducer is rotated 90 degrees to obtain the sagittal plane and is then tilted from right to left on the anterior fontanelle (Fig. 93.2a). It is suggested that each examiner establish a standard sequence of obtaining the images to avoid any mislabelling of the laterality.

For instance, one can make it a habit to search for pathologic changes by proceeding from the left hemisphere across

the midline to the right hemisphere. Beginning with the midline section, as seen on Figure 93.2c, review once more the normal topographic anatomy of the sagittal hemispheric sections. It is important to confirm the regular appearance of the corpus callosum (126) and overlying cingulate gyrus (130). The cerebellum (110) appears as a hyperechoic structure behind the pons (145) in the posterior cerebral fossa (see Fig. 94.2).

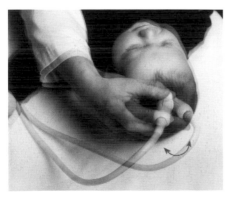

Fig. 93.2 a

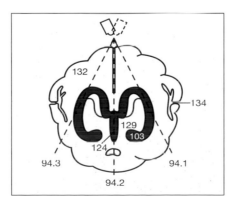

Fig. 93.2 b

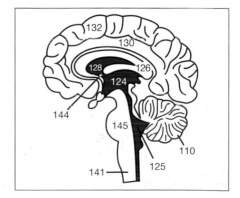

Fig. 93.2 c

Sagittal Sections

The thalamus **(129)** is in the center of the oblique, laterally tilted sections (**Figs. 94.1** and **94.3**). The anechoic CSF in the lateral ventricle **(103)** is located above, containing the hyperechoic choroid plexus **(104)**, which should have a smooth contour without local bulging (DD: choroid plexus hemorrhage, see page 96). If the corpus callosum **(126)** is normally developed, the cerebral sulci **(133)** of the parietal and occipital lobes do not extend to the lateral ventricles and terminate instead along the cingulate gyrus **(130)**.

Figure 94.1 shows an oblique angulated sagittal section through the left lateral ventricle. A midline section including pons **(145)**, hyperechoic cerebellum **(110)** and 4th ventricle **(125)** is shown in **Figure 94.2**.

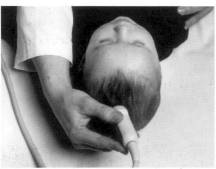

Fig. 94.1 a

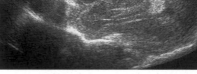

Fig. 94.1 b

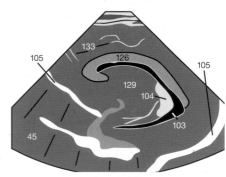

Fig. 94.1 c

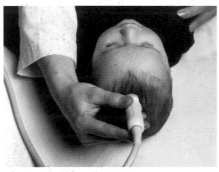

Fig. 94.2 a

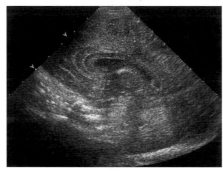

Fig. 94.2 b

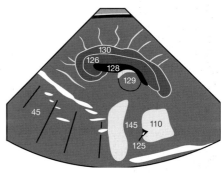

Fig. 94.2 c

Choroid Plexus Cysts

Unilateral, small choroid plexus cysts **(64)** can represent normal variants (**Fig. 94.3**). The presumed cause is above all small prenatal hemorrhages, but prenatal viral infections are also discussed. If the cyst is small and does not impair the CSF circulation, it generally has no clinical consequence. Only larger CSF-filled defects in the cerebral parenchyma ("porencephaly") suggest areas of resorption following larger hemorrhages or malformation anomalies.

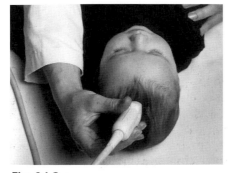

Fig. 94.3 a

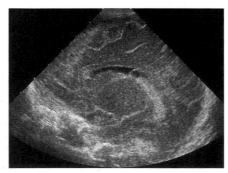

Fig. 94.3 b

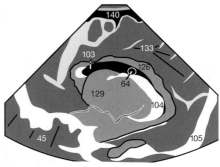

Fig. 94.3 c

Premature Newborns

The normal cerebral sulci can be totally absent in preterm newborns delivered around the 28th gestational week. In general, the sonographically apparent cerebral gyration is less in preterm than in term newborns, without indicating any underlying maturation disturbance. Consequently, the neonatal CSF spaces are more capacious and partially asymmetric (Fig. 95.2).

Furthermore, preterm newborns also can have an incompletely developed corpus callosum, seen as a thin hypoechoic line just above the cavum septi pellucidi on the coronal section. Only follow-up examinations can distinguish physiologic immaturity from impaired CSF flow or a genuine hypo- or aplastic corpus callosum (Fig. 95.3).

Cavum Septi Pellucidi

Incomplete fusion of the two laminae of the septum pellucidum between the frontal horns leads to a CSF-filled cavum septi pellucidi (128), which usually obliterates within the first months of life but persists into adulthood in about 20% of cases (Fig. 95.1). A more occipitally located CSF-containing slitlike space is referred to as cavum vergae.

Slight asymmetry of the lateral ventricles (103) is another normal variant without underlying obstruction to the CSF flow. Figure 95.2 shows a wide anechoic CSF space lateral to the choroid plexus (104), but only on the left and absent on the right (the coronal images are viewed from the front, with resultant reversal of the hemispheres).

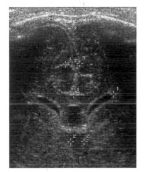

Fig. 95.1 a

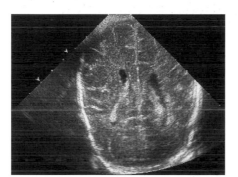

Fig. 95.2 a

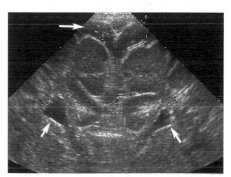

Fig. 95.3 a

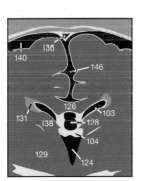

Fig. 95.1 b

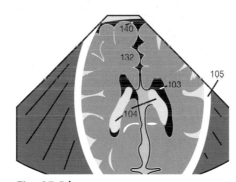

Fig. 95.2 b

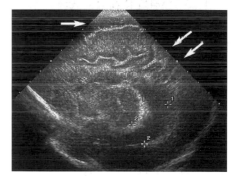

Fig. 95.3 b

Agenesis of the Corpus Callosum

The corpus callosum is involved in many developmental disorders, syndromes and inborn metabolic errors, but can also be affected by hypoxia or infections. The spectrum of callosal abnormalities ranges from partial to complete (agenesis) absence of the corpus callosum. On the coronal section (Fig. 95.3a), agenesis of the corpus callosum leads to a "steer horn" appearance of both frontal horns (↗ ↖), which are widely spaced to each other and more laterally located than usual.

The sagittal section (Fig. 95.3b) shows no cingulate sulcus (Fig. 94.1) and resultant radiation of the cerebral sulci to the lateral ventricles (↙ ↙), making it easy to recognize even a partial agenesis of the corpus callosum. The case shown in Figure 95.3 has not only prominent lateral ventricles but also a prominent subarachnoidal CSF space (➡) as part of a diffuse cerebral atrophy (Fig. 93.1).

Pathophysiology

The ventricles are lined by the so-called ependyma. The subependymal germinal matrix, which proliferates between the 24th and 32nd gestational week with corresponding high vascularity, is located beneath the ependymal lining. During the period of rapid growth, the germinal matrix is very sensitive to blood pressure fluctuations, since the mechanism for regulating intracerebral blood flow is not yet fully developed.

This transient fetal anatomy has been implicated in the pathogenesis of neonatal cerebral hemorrhage in the subependymal region and around the choroid plexus. According to the severity, the hemorrhage is classified into four grades as listed in the adjacent table.

Neonatal Cerebral Hemorrhage – Grading	
Grade 1	Isolated subependymal hemorrhage
Grade 2	Subependymal hemorrhage with ventricular extension (involving less than 50% of the ventricular lumen) without ventricular dilation
Grade 3	Intraventricular hemorrhage (involving more than 50% of the ventricular lumen) and ventricular dilation
Grade 4	Additional extension into the cerebral parenchyma

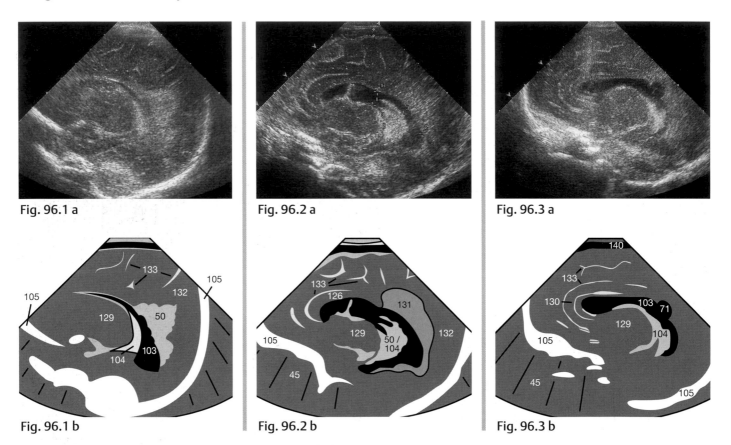

Fig. 96.1 a   Fig. 96.2 a   Fig. 96.3 a

Fig. 96.1 b   Fig. 96.2 b   Fig. 96.3 b

Sonographic Findings

Acute hemorrhage (50) is hyperechoic in comparison to the cerebral parenchyma (132) and usually located in the vicinity of the ventricles (Fig. 96.1) for the pathophysiologic reasons outlined above. An irregularly shaped or bulging choroid plexus (104) suggests a hemorrhage (50) in the plexus (Fig. 96.2).

Following an earlier intrauterine hemorrhage, the resorbed blood leaves behind CSF-filled parenchymal defects (71) that can be mistaken for ventricular dilation (103) (Fig. 96.3). Therefore, the differential diagnosis between periventricular parenchymal defect and genuine hydrocephalus will be discussed on the next page.

Hydrocephalus

An obstructive (internal) hydrocephalus (Fig. 97.1) is usually caused by blood-induced subarachnoidal adhesions that block the normal CSF outflow. Less frequent causes include compression of CSF pathways by an aneurysm of the vein of Galen, a biconvex (!) cyst of the septum pellucidum (compare with cavum septi pellucidi, Fig. 95.1) blocking the foramen of Monro, or an aqueduct stenosis. Blocked foramina of Luschka and Magendie added to an aqueduct stenosis can cause an isolated dilation of the 4th ventricle.

The resultant increased intraventricular pressure will first enlarge and expand the temporal horns, since they are met by the lowest resistance of the surrounding cerebral parenchyma. Only later (Fig. 97.1), the entire lateral ventricles dilate and expand with corresponding narrowing of the subarachnoidal CSF spaces. The increased pressure must be relieved by a shunt (↖ in Fig. 97.2).

A long-standing hydrocephalus should be relieved slowly, since a rapid drop in pressure puts tension on the external cerebral vessels to tension (risk of hemorrhage). After a shunt has been placed, follow-up examinations are indicated to check the position of the shunt and to exclude malfunction of the shunt valve.

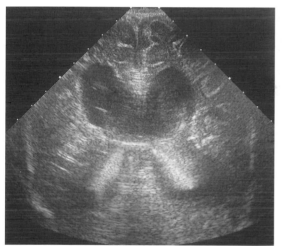

Fig. 97.1

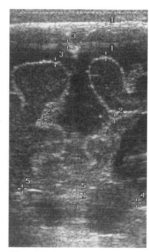

Fig. 97.3 a

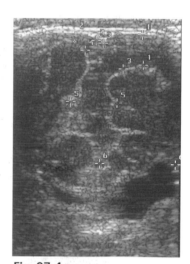

Fig. 97.4 a

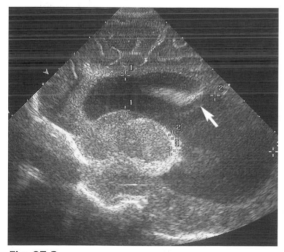

Fig. 97.2

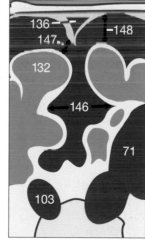

Fig. 97.3 b

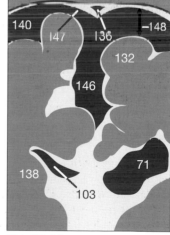

Fig. 97.4 b

Cerebral Atrophy

The width of the subarachnoidal CSF spaces allows a differentiation between obstructive (internal) hydrocephalus and an enlarged ventricular system due to cerebral atrophy. The imaging should be done with a linear transducer because of its better near-field resolution. Figure 97.3 shows definite widening of the CSF space in diffuse cerebral atrophy involving both hemispheres (Fig. 93.1). Please note the unusually good visualization of the superior sagittal sinus (136). Unilateral parenchymal defects (71) widen the ipsilateral subarachnoidal CSF spaces (148) in comparison to the other side (Fig. 97.4). Moreover, the superficial cerebral sulci appear rather prominent in cerebral atrophy and are more effaced in hydrocephalus.

P

Checking the Shunt Valve System in Hydrocephalus

When malfunction of the CSF shunt is sonographically suspected, e.g., continuing progression of the ventricular enlargement, the examiner should check not only the correct intraventricular position of the shunt tip (**Fig. 97.2**) but also the continuity of remaining shunt catheter.

The adjacent radiographs of a shunt series show a disconnected (✎) valve (**Fig. 98.1a**) that has been reconnected after shunt revision (**Fig. 98.1b**). With the growth of the child, shunts may need to be replaced or revised.

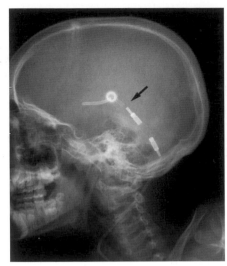

Fig. 98.1 a

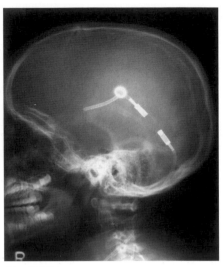

Fig. 98.1 b

Spinal Canal

In the newborn, the conus medullaris (142) of the spinal cord (141) is visualized from the back with a 5.0 to 7.5 MHz transducer on the prone patient (**Fig. 98.2**). The spinal cord is demarcated form the anechoic spinal CSF space (140) by a delicate hyperechoic line representing the pia mater. The hyperechoic double line in the center of the cord does not correspond to the central canal, but to the interface between the white commissure and the anterior median fissure.

The roots of the cauda equina (143) extend caudally, accounting for the hyperechoic structure around the conus, which should not extend below the L 2/3 disc space in the newborn.

For the localization of the sacrum, it is helpful to remember that S1 protrudes posteriorly from the straight vertebral line posteriorly (toward the transducer).

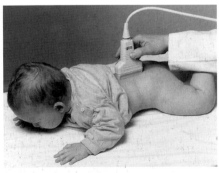

Fig. 98.2 a

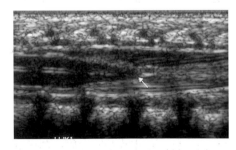

Fig. 98.2 b

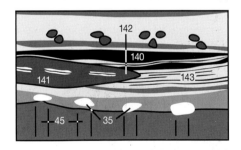

Fig. 98.2 c

When increasing ossification of the vertebral arches limits the delineation of the spinal canal, the evaluation has to be done with magnetic resonance imaging (MRI). The M-mode can document the important observation of free oscillation of the cord synchronously with respiration and cardiac rate.

Absent pulsation, distortion or low position of the conus and fixation of the cord to the spinal canal indicate a tethered cord, which often is primarily caused by an intraspinal lipoma or epidermoid cyst. A tethered cord can also be acquired as postsurgical cicatricial fixation of neural structures.

Anatomy

The thyroid gland is examined with a 7.5 MHz linear transducer. With the head slightly extended, transverse sections of the thyroid gland are systematically obtained in the craniocaudal direction (**Fig. 99.1a**). Thereafter, sagittal sections are obtained through each thyroid lobe (**Fig. 99.1b**). A general orientation for the transverse sections is provided by the midline acoustic shadowing of the trachea (**84**) and, farther laterally, by the anechoic crosssections of the carotid arteries (**82**) and jugular veins (**83**). The thyroid parenchyma (**81**) is situated between the vessels and trachea. A thin parenchymal band (isthmus) connects both thyroid lobes (**Fig. 99.2**) anterior to the trachea. The carotid artery (**82**) usually is posteromedially located, and appears round and incompressible in the transverse plane. The jugular vein (**83**) is more anterolaterally located, has a typical biphasic venous pulse and is compressible with graded (!) pressure applied to the transducer.

For any uncertainty with the assignment of the vascular structures, the patient can be asked to perform a Valsalva maneuver (bearing down with the vocal chords closed). The induced venous blockage distends the jugular veins, allowing easy anatomic orientation. The normal thyroid parenchyma (**81**) is slightly more echogenic (brighter) than the more anteriorly located sternohyoideus (**89**) and sternothyroideus (**90**) muscle and the more laterally located sternocleidomastoideus (**85**) muscle (**Fig. 99.2**).

Volumetry

To determine the volume of the thyroid gland, maximum transverse and sagittal (anteroposterior) diameters of each lobe are measured on transverse sections. These values are multiplied by the maximum length as measured on the sagittal sections and the product is multiplied by 0.5. Within an error range of approximately 10%, the result corresponds to the volume (in ml) of each lobe. The volume of the thyroid gland should not exceed 25 ml in men and 18 ml in women (see Table on page 101).

Small cysts (**64**) in the thyroid gland (**81**) might not cause any distal acoustic enhancement (**Fig. 99.3b**) and must be differentiated from hypoechoic nodules and cross-sectioned vessels.

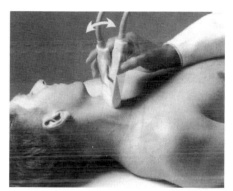

Fig. 99.1 a

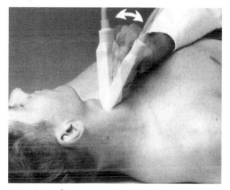

Fig. 99.1 b

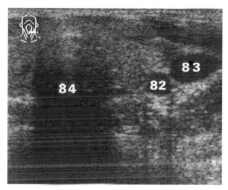

Fig. 99.1 c

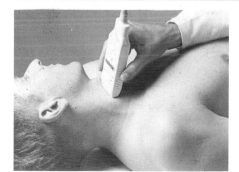

Fig. 99.2 a

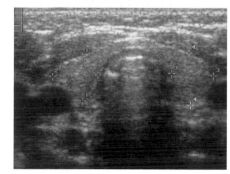

Fig. 99.2 b

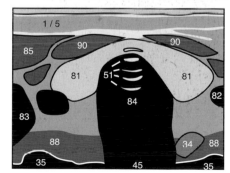

Fig. 99.2 c

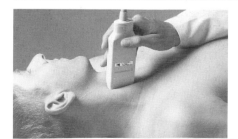

Fig. 99.3 a

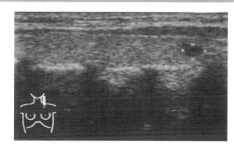

Fig. 99.3 b

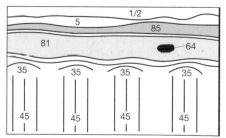

Fig. 99.3 c

Goiter

In iodine-deficient geographic areas, the most common diffuse thyroid condition is iodine deficiency goiter, e.g., a diffuse enlargement of the thyroid gland. Compared to their normal appearance **(Fig. 99.2)**, both thyroid lobes are enlarged and expanded **(Fig. 100.2)**, often with a thickened isthmus. The iodine deficiency frequently induces isoechoic nodules (↙) in the struma, which, if located peripherally, produce a nodularly protruding organ surface **(Fig. 100.3)**. With time, regressive calcifications or cysts (64 in **Fig. 100.4**) frequently develop in these nodules (54). Through continuing degeneration, the anechoic cysts can reach a considerable size **(Fig. 100.5)** and can centrally show hyperechoic hemorrhagic foci **(↘ in Fig. 100.6)**.

Malignant degeneration of hyperechoic or isoechoic nodules is very rare (in the per mille range). Hypoechoic thyroid nodules are different (see next page).

Fig. 100.1

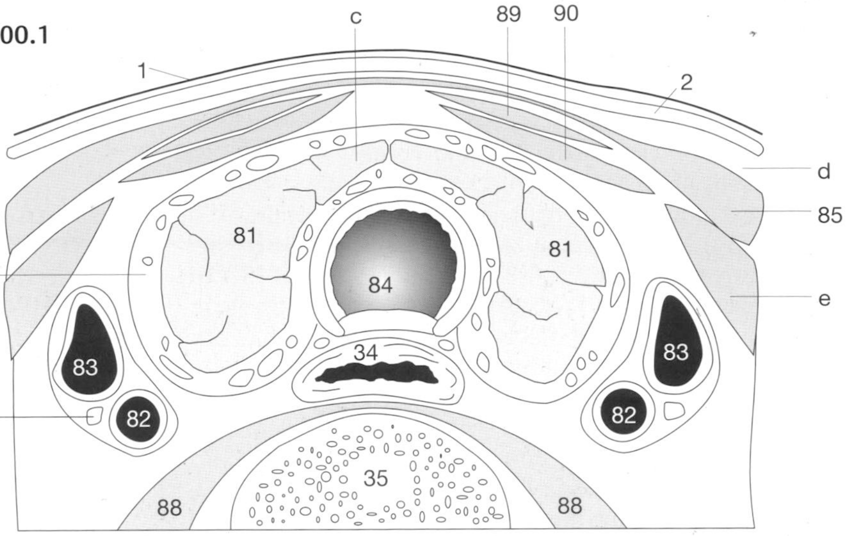

Anatomy of the thyroid region

(a) vagus nerve
(b) fibrous capsule of thyroid
(c) isthmus
(d) platysma
(e) omohyoid muscle
(1) skin
(2) subcutaneous fat tissue
(34) esophagus
(35) spine
(81) lateral lobes of thyroid
(82) common carotid artery
(83) internal jugular vein
(84) trachea
(85) sternocleidomastoid muscle
(88) anterior scalenus muscle and medial scalenus muscle
(89) sternohyoid muscle
(90) sternothyroid muscle

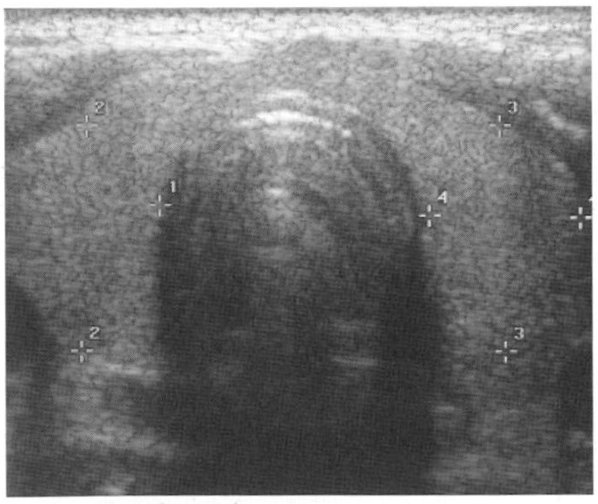

Fig. 100.2

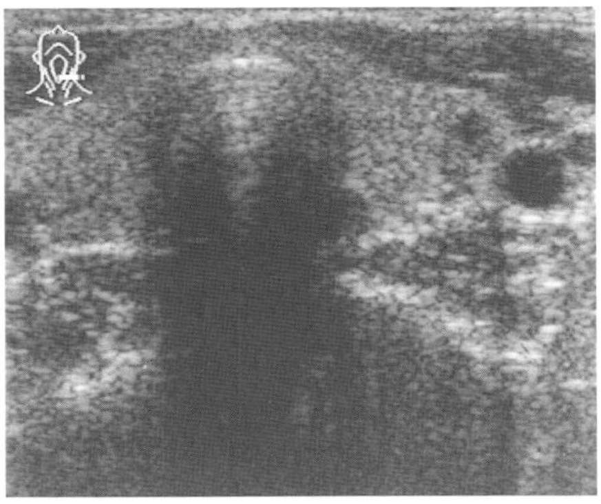

Fig. 100.4 a

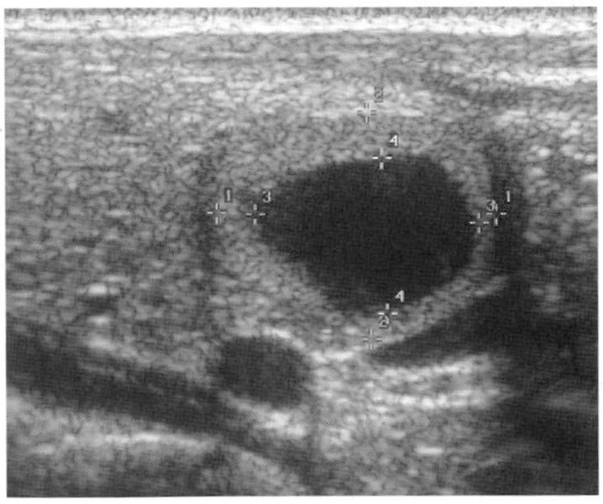

Fig. 100.5

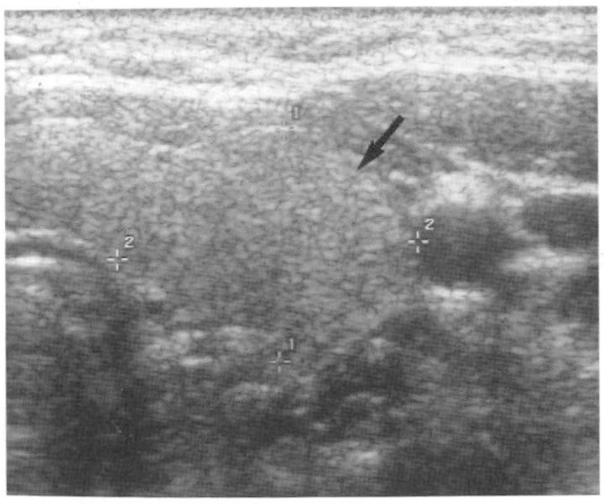

Fig. 100.3

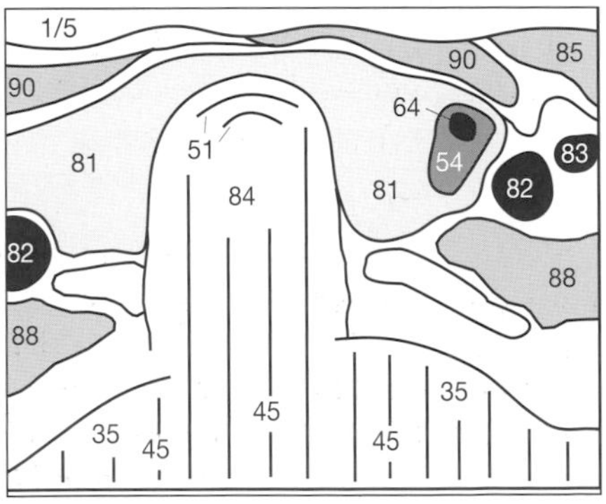

Fig. 100.4 b

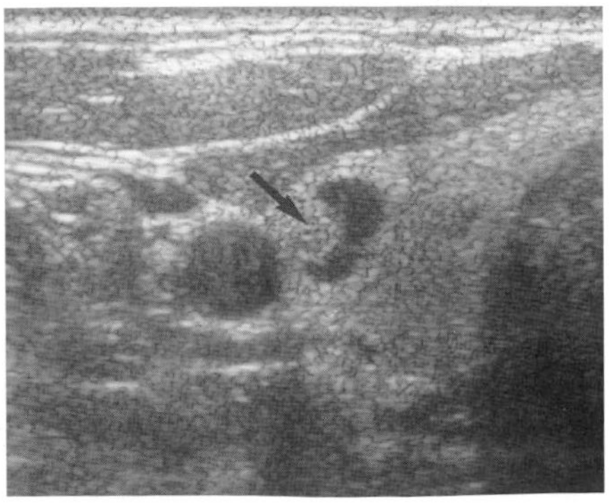

Fig. 100.6

Focal, Solid Nodules

The differential diagnosis of hypoechoic thyroid lesions includes cystic degeneration and benign adenomas, but also thyroid carcinomas.

Scintigraphically functioning ("hot") nodules are hormone-producing adenomas **(72)** and frequently appear sonographically with a hypoechoic rim amidst the normal thyroid parenchyma **(81) (Fig. 101.1)**. In the thyroid gland, a hypoechoic rim (halo) does **not** indicate malignancy, which is in contrast to the typical sonographic morphology of hepatic metastases (see page 40).

Scintigraphically non-functioning ("cold") and sonographically hypoechoic **nodules (54)** need further evaluation, e.g., needle aspiration for cytology or biopsy, to exclude a malignancy **(Fig. 101.2)**.

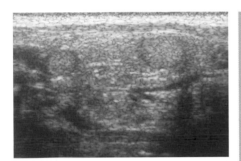

Fig. 101.1 a

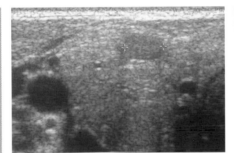

Fig. 101.2 a

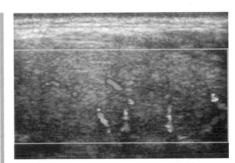

Fig. 101.3

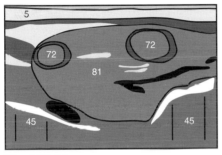

Fig. 101.1 b

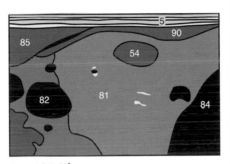

Fig. 101.2 b

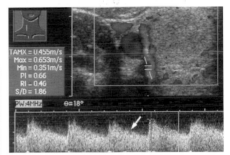

Fig. 101.4

Thyroiditis

The autoimmune ("Hashimoto") thyroiditis is diffusely hypoechoic relative to the normally more hyperechoic thyroid parenchyma. The hypoechogenicity is caused by chronic lymphocytic infiltration and, in contrast to Graves disease, persists for life. In addition, the echo texture appears coarse and heterogeneous, and contains an increase in hyperperfused vessels **(Fig. 101.3)**.

The M-mode (time display of the blood flow) of supplemental color Doppler sonography **(Fig. 101.4)** shows hyperperfusion with increased flow level during diastole (✎).

The subacute ("de Quervain") thyroiditis is characterized by thyroid enlargement with indistinctly outlined hypoechoic areas within zones of normal echogenicity.

Thyroid Gland – Volumetry

Nutritional iodine intake must be considered when establishing normal values for the thyroid volume measured by ultrasound. In countries with iodine deficiency, e.g., Germany, the "normal values" are higher than the expected physiologic normative data.

Normal Values of the Thyroid Volume

Girls younger than 15 years have a slightly higher thyroid volume than boys. Considering the dependence of iodine nutrition on the thyroid size, the upper limits are listed separately for iodine deficiency (black numbers) and for adequate iodine intake (blue numbers).

Age	Females	Males
Newborns	< 2.3 (1.5)	< 3.5 (2.0)
1 – 4 years	< 4.7 (3.0)	< 3.8 (2.9)
5 – 10 years	< 6.5 (5.0)	< 6.0 (5.4)
11 – 12 years	< 14.6 (14.1)	< 13.9 (13.2)
Adults	< 18.0	< 25.0

The blue numbers in parenthesis represent the normal values for children living in countries **without** iodine deficiency. The highest thyroid volumes accepted as normal are listed here for both lobes together, calculated according to the volume formula 0.5 x A x B x C. The mean volumes are considerably lower.

Enlarged lymph nodes (55) show up as oval hypoechoic space-occupying lesions and are often located in vicinity of the cervical neurovascular bundle (Fig. 102.1), along the internal jugular vein (83) and carotid artery (82), but are also found submentally. Lymph nodes that are reactively enlarged as part of a viral or bacterial infection are usually elongated, with the ratio of the longitudinal diameter divided by the transverse diameter (the L/T ratio) exceeding 2.0, and can appear in groups (Fig. 102.2). A further sign indicating physiologic nodal enlargement is a centrally located hyperechoic hilum (Fig. 102.3) with a prominent hilar vascular pattern (= hilus sign).

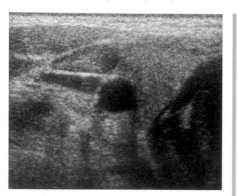

Fig. 102.1 a

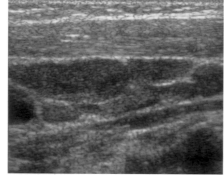

Fig. 102.2 a

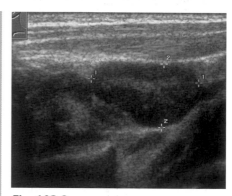

Fig. 102.3 a

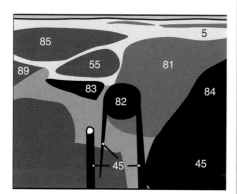

Fig. 102.1 b

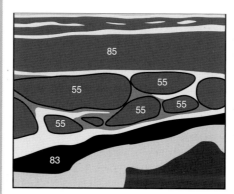

Fig. 102.2 b

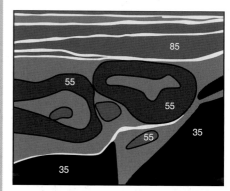

Fig. 102.3 b

In contrast, plump, spherical lymph nodes with an L/T ratio around 1.0 and without a hilar sign are suspicious for pathologic nodal enlargement (lymphoma / metastasis). If the nature of nodal enlargement remains in doubt after applying the above-mentioned criteria, color duplex sonography (Fig. 102.4b) should be considered before an excisional biopsy. Lymphomas frequently exhibit a diffuse perfusion pattern with branching perfusion toward the periphery instead of the normal perfusion toward the hilum.

Especially in children, a possible abscess with anechoic liquefaction (↖) should be looked for (Fig. 102.4a), since nodal abscess is an indication for surgical intervention. The center of the liquefaction lacks any perfused vessels on color duplex sonography.

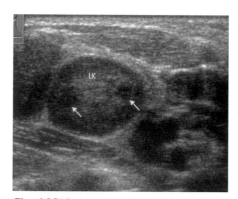

Fig. 102.4 a

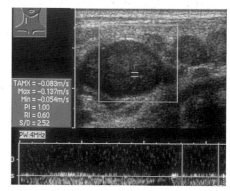

Fig. 102.4 b

Benign vs. Malignant Lymph Nodes

Criteria	Benign	Malignant
Ratio length / width	> 2.0	~ 1.0
Hilus sign	Positive	Negative
Vascularization	Centered in the hilus	Diffuse or branching

Here are a few questions for the head and neck region. You will find the answers on the preceding pages. The answer to the image question is on page 109.

1. Topic hydrocephaly: Please list here all five normal values for the internal and subarachnoidal CSF spaces in the term newborn. What do the common acronyms for the respective measurements stand for (compound terms)?

Acronym	Compound term	Upper normal value for term newborns
CSW		< mm
CCW		< mm
IHW		< mm
LVW		< mm
3rd VW		< mm

2. Draw a sketch of the adjacent **Figure 103.1** that copies it as exactly as possible and annotate each anatomic detail you recognize on the image. Thereafter, add to the sketch where and at what angle you would have measured the external subarachnoidal CSF spaces and ventricles (see question 1). Finally, you should consider which normal variant is present in this sample image.

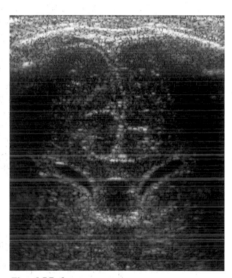

Fig. 103.1 a

Fig. 103.1 b

3. What criteria do you know for distinguishing between benign and malignant enlargement of lymph nodes? List at least 3 criteria for physiologic and malignant nodal enlargement.

Benign Criteria	Malignant Criteria

4. How do benign thyroid adenomas typically (not necessarily) appear? What criteria taken together are suspicious for thyroid malignancy?

Q

P

Correct Positioning

To exclude a developmental dysplasia of the hip, the baby must lie exactly 90 degrees on the side, placed in a hip board device designed by Graf (**Fig. 104.1a**). The examiner holds the upper leg in slight flexion with one hand. Extending the hip does not offer any advantage for finding the correct image plane and often irritates the baby. The infant shown here has the hip flexed too much. The knee should not lie on top of the hip board.

Finding the Correct Image Plane

The transducer must be placed strictly aligned along the lateromedial plane, with the ilium (112) exactly horizontal and sharply outlined in the image plane (**Fig. 104.1b**). From the anechoic acetabular promontory (159), the medial osseous acetabular roof (160) extends as a hyperechoic line away from the transducer (**Fig. 104.1**). The lateral cartilaginous portion of the acetabular roof extends toward the transducer and terminates at the acetabular labrum (158). When the maximal size of the femoral head (153) is centered and the ossification centers of the femoral neck (162) appear sharply demarcated, you have found the correct imaging plane.

The Y cartilage of the acetabulum (164) is seen as anechoic interruption of the ilium (161) at the lower edge of the image. Most examiners prefer the image orientation shown here (left image border = cranial). The 90-degree rotated or reversed display was customary in the past, but no longer corresponds to the general guidelines and is selected much less often.

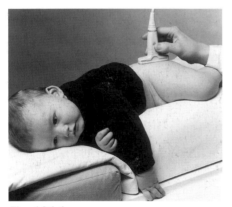

Fig. 104.1 a

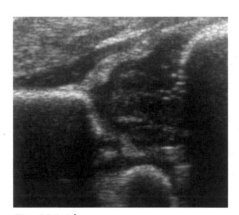

Fig. 104.1 b

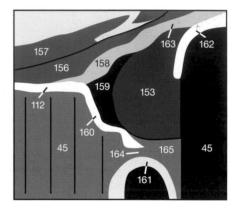

Fig. 104.1 c

Angle Measurements

First, the longitudinal axis (---) is marked along the ilium (112) (**Figs. 104.2/3**). Then the tangent to the promontory along the osseous acetabular roof is added. The alpha (α) angle is measured between both lines. It exceeds 60 degrees in mature hips. Smaller angles should be confirmed by repeating the measurements several times; if they are reproducible, this suggests a dysplasia.

The subsequent measurement of the beta (β) angle is subject to a greater error, since exact positioning through the acetabular labrum (158) often proves difficult. The beta angle should normally measure less than 55 degrees (see next page). The prescribed magnification is 1.7, but it has become customary to take the measurements on images magnified by a factor or 2.0 to 2.5 (**Fig. 104.4**).

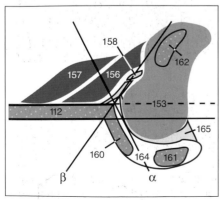

Fig. 104.2

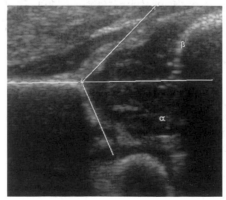

Fig. 104.3

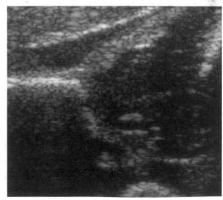

Fig. 104.4

Classification of Infant Hips According to Graf

In developmental dysplasia of the hip, the femoral head (∗) increasingly migrates superolaterally. On the radiograph **(Fig. 105.2)**, the osseous acetabular roof is no longer close to the horizontal line (➡) and instead is inclined more superiorly (↗) in lateral direction. The MRI **(Fig. 105.3)** illustrates an extreme case of a completely dislocated femoral head (∗) and an empty acetabulum (↘) that is obvious in comparison with the contralateral side. The sonographically determined alpha angle decreases with increasing severity of the dysplasia.

As a rule of thumb, the alpha angle should be larger than 60 degrees after the first year of life at the latest. However, only an alpha angle of more than 63 degrees can exclude dysplasia with certainty. If the hip remains a sonographic

Classification of Infant Hips according to Graf	Alpha	Beta	Femoral head
I (normal)	> 60°	< 55°	centered
II a+	56 – 59°	55 – 70°	centered
II a-	50 – 55°	55 – 70°	centered
II g	44 – 49°	55 – 77°	centered
II d	44 – 49°	> 77°	centered
III (eccentric)	< 44°	> 77°	eccentric
IV (dislocated)	< 44°	undetermined	dislocated

type II a beyond the second month of life, a growth disturbance must be considered and wide diapers are recommended. Persistence of these changes for the next 4 to 8 weeks or an alpha angle less than 50 degrees is an indication for therapy with splint devices.

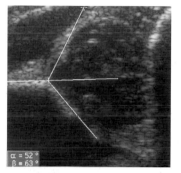

Fig. 105.1

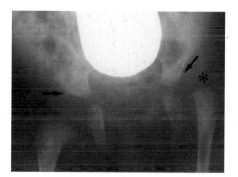

Fig. 105.2

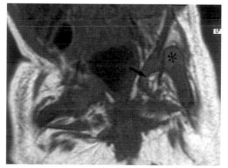

Fig. 105.3

Transient Synovitis of the Hip

Thickened synovia and joint effusion are typical findings of acquired hip diseases. The supine child is examined with an anteriorly placed high-frequency linear transducer **(Fig. 105.4a)**. The normal joint space (168) appears as thin anechoic space between hyperechoic joint capsule (163) and the anterior contour of the femoral epiphysis (166) and metaphysis (167) **(Fig. 105.4b)**. The indentation of the femoral epiphyseal plate (107) is easily recognized.

Measuring the height of the epiphysis (⬅➡) on serial follow-up examinations can easily establish a loss of height, e.g., as occurring in necrosis of the femoral head.

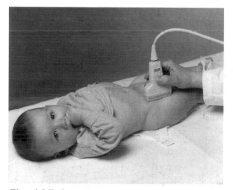

Fig. 105.4 a

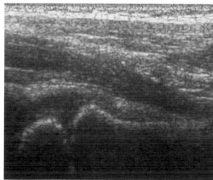

Fig. 105.4 b

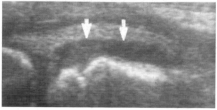

Fig. 105.4 c

A transient joint effusion frequently develops as part of a viral infection and is seen as anechoic widening (⬇⬇) of the joint space **(Fig. 105.5)**. A joint effusion that lasts longer than two weeks or an edematous, anechoic thickening of the joint capsule suggests Legg-Calvé-Perthes disease or septic arthritis and should be further evaluated by MRI.

Fig. 105.5

Answer to Fig. 16.4:

The image shows a longitudinal section of the aorta (15). Its wall contains hyper-echoic calcifications = atherosclerotic plaques (49) with posterior acoustic shadows (45). Without acoustic shadowing, the larger plaques could have been easily overlooked since they are located just next to hyperechoic (= bright) intestinal air (46), which also induces acoustic shadows. Furthermore, the image shows below (= posterior to) the aorta (15) the phenomenon of posterior sound enhancement (70).

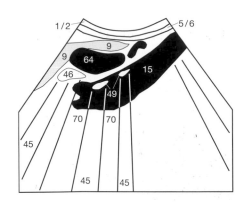

Fig. 106.1

Answer to Fig. 17.1:

In preparation for the practical sessions, the student should become familiar with spatial orientation in a three-dimensional space. To make the first step easy, only two planes perpendicular to each other should be considered: the vertical (sagittal) plane (**Fig. 106.2**) and the horizontal (transverse) plane (**Fig. 106.3**).

As suggested on page 17, a coffee filter can help to picture how the sound waves propagate through the body in these two planes from the anteriorly placed transducer. Both planes display the anterior abdominal wall at the upper image border (superior aspect of the image = anterior). Since by convention all sagittal sections are viewed as seen from the patient's right side (**Fig. 106.2a**), the superiorly located patient structures are displayed at the left image border (left side of the image = superior) and the inferiorly located structures at the right image border.

The transverse plane is displayed after the transducer is rotated 90 degrees. Since this plane is viewed from below, the display of the visualized structures is inverted (left = right) (**Fig. 106.3b**). This orientation conforms to the customary display of CT and MRI. Standing in front of the patient, the liver, for instance, is also seen on the left. Therefore, this display makes sense. The only exception is that neurosurgeons view the cranial CT from above, since this corresponds to the neurosurgical intraoperative approach.

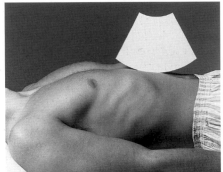

Fig. 106.2 a

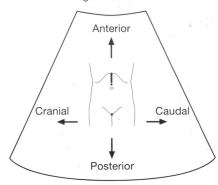

Fig. 106.2 b

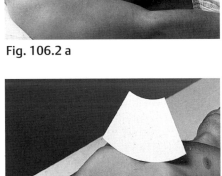

Fig. 106.3 a

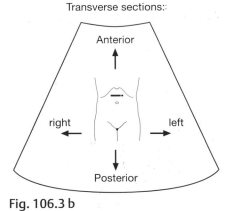

Fig. 106.3 b

Answers to Fig.18.4 – 18.6:

The three images have in common that the structures on the far left are less well delineated than usual – the image in **Figure 18.4** appears indistinct and is diffusely superimposed with scattered sound waves. This is caused by inadequate pressure applied to the transducer, which is a typical mistake made by a novice, and not by a lack of gel.

If the amount of gel actually is inadequate or the examiner loses skin coupling by tilting the transducer, an image as shown in **Figure 18.5** is produced. A black band is seen along

the margin of the lost skin coupling (here on the right side of the image). It immediately begins at the skin-transducer interface and not at a certain depth, which distinguishes lost skin coupling from acoustic shadows behind ribs, intestinal air, gallstones and renal calculi. The image shown in **Figure 18.6** was obtained on the same patient a few second later after improved skin coupling and properly applied pressure on the transducer – all structures are much better seen.

Answer to Fig. 24.2 (Question 7):

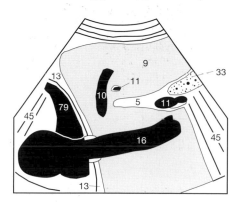

Answer to Fig. 32.1 (Question 4):

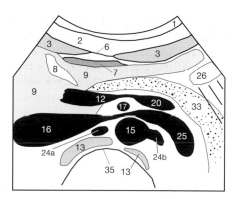

Answer to Fig. 44.1 (Question 5):

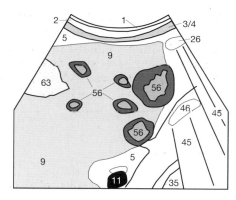

Sonographic section:
Sagittal section of the upper abdomen, paramedian over the inferior vena cava (16)
Organs:
Liver (9), heart and pancreas (33)
Structures:
Diaphragm (13), hepatic vein (10), portal branch (11), caudate lobe (9a)
Significant finding:
Anechoic space (79) between myo-/epicardium and diaphragm
Diagnosis: Pericardial effusion (79)
Differential diagnosis: Epicardial fat

Sonographic section: Sagittal section of the upper abdomen at the level of the renal vein crossing
Organs: Liver (9), stomach (26), pancreas (33)
Vessels: Aorta (15), IVC (16), renal artery (24), renal vein (25), superior mesenteric artery (17), confluence (12)
Structures: Ligaments (7, 8), rectus muscle (3), lumbar vertebra (35)
Significant finding:
Prominent lumen of the renal vein (25)
Diagnosis: Still physiologic, no pathologic dilation of the left renal vein (due to "nutcracker" effect between 15 and 17)

Sonographic section:
Right oblique subcostal section
Organs: Liver (9), stomach (26), small bowel (46)
Significant finding:
Homogeneous hyperechoic, sharply demarcated area (63); multiple round to oval intrahepatic lesions with hypo-echoic rim
Diagnosis:
Focal fatty infiltration (63) and multiple hepatic metastases (56) – at least two episodes of metastatic spreading, since new and older metastatic foci are visible next to each other

Answer to Fig. 44.2 (Question 5):

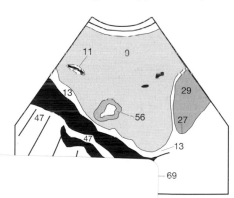

Answer to Fig. 44.3 (Question 5):

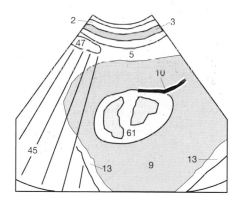

Answer to Fig. 44.4 (Question 7):

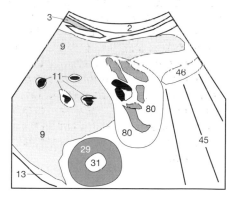

right

29), lung (47)
ıatic hepatic
ıechoic rim

ımangioma
ıicity, but the

Sonographic section: Sagittal section of the right upper quadrant of the abdomen along the paramedian plane
Organs: Liver (9), lung (47), diaphragm (13)
Significant finding: Hyperechoic, partially heterogeneous space-occupying intrahepatic lesion
Diagnosis: Hemangioma (61) with draining vein (10)
Differential diagnosis: Hyperechoic metastasis, hepatic tumors of other origin

Sonographic section: Oblique subcostal section of the right upper quadrant of the abdomen
Organs: Liver (9), gallbladder (80), kidney (29)
Significant finding: Heterogeneous, poorly demarcated abnormality at the inferior hepatic border
Diagnosis: Cholecystitis with marked wall thickening (80)
Differential diagnosis: Parasitic involvement of liver or gallbladder, sludge, bowel content

Answer to Fig. 62.1 (Question 6):

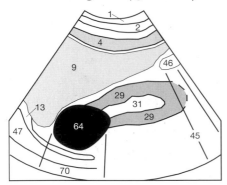

Sonographic section:
Intercostal plane of the right flank
Organs: Liver (**9**),
kidney (**29**), lung (**47**), bowel (**46**)
Structures:
Diaphragm (**13**), renal pelvis (**31**)
Significant finding:
Anechoic, spherical and sharply
demarcated lesion (**64**) at the upper
pole of the right kidney, with posterior
sound enhancement (**70**)
Diagnosis: Renal cyst (**64**)
Differential diagnosis: Adrenal tumor
with cystic component

Answer to Fig. 62.2 (Question 6):

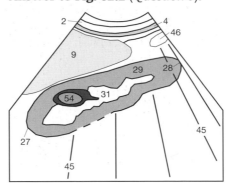

Sonographic section:
Intercostal plane of the right flank
in left lateral decubitus position
Organs: Liver (**9**), bowel (**46**) with
acoustic shadowing (**45**), kidney (**29**)
Structures:
Oblique abdominal muscles (**4**), upper
renal pole (**27**), lower renal pole (**28**)
Significant finding:
Hypoechoic tumor (**54**) in the renal
parenchyma (**29**) with space-occupy-
ing effect and sharp demarcation
Diagnosis: Renal cell carcinoma
Differential diagnosis: Renal lympho-
ma, metastasis, hyperplastic column
of Bertini, hemorrhagic renal cyst

Answer to Fig. 62.3 (Question 7):

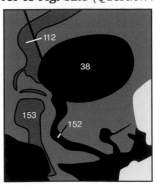

This radiographic image of a voiding
cystourethrogram was obtained during
voiding (urethra = **152**), with the
patient slightly oblique for better
visualization of the prevesical ureter in
case of ureteral reflux.

The dark line extending upward
from the urinary bladder (**38**)
represents the obliquely visualized
cortex of the ilium (**112**) projected on
the femoral head (**153**). This visualized
part of a normal ilium should not be
mistaken for a retrograde filled ureter
as manifestation of reflux.

Answer to Fig. 62.4 (Question 9):

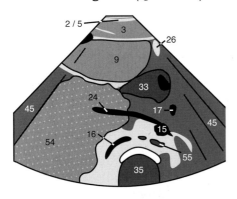

Sonographic section:
Transverse section of the right upper
quadrant of the abdomen in an infant
Organs: Liver (**9**), pancreas (**33**)
Significant finding:
Poorly demarcated organs; large heterogeneous tumor (**54**), paravertebrally
on the right, with anterior displacement
of the right renal artery (**24**); suspicious
for nodal metastasis (**55**) between
aorta (**15**) and lumbar vertebra (**35**)
Diagnosis:
Metastatic nephroblastoma (**54**)
Differential diagnosis: Neuroblastoma
of the right sympathetic chain

Answer to Fig. 72.1 (Question 5):

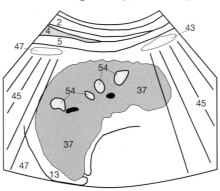

Sonographic section:
High section of the left flank in the
right lateral decubitus position
Organs: Spleen (**37**), lung (**47**),
colon (**43**), diaphragm (**13**)
Significant finding:
Several homogeneously hyperechoic
lesions (**54**) in the splenic parenchyma,
without hyperechoic rim
Diagnosis (rare finding):
Multiple splenic hemangiomas
Differential diagnosis:
Hyperechoic metastases, vasculitis as
part of systemic lupus erythematosus,
histiocytosis X

Answer to Fig. 90.1 (Question 7):

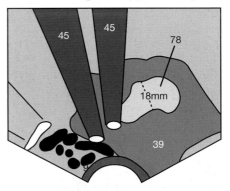

Sonographic section:
Endovaginal view of the uterus
Organs:
Uterus (**39**)
Significant finding:
Up to about 18-mm width of the hete-
rogeneous, hyperechoic endometrium
(**78**), in a menopausal woman without
hormonal therapy (see question)
Diagnosis:
Suspicious for endometrial carcinoma;
work-up: fractionated D and C and
histologic confirmation

Answer to Question on Page 40

These are the artifacts of "posterior sound enhancement" (70) and "edge effect" (45) behind the gallbladder (14). Figure 37.3a shows two pathologic fluids:

68 = ascites below the diaphragm
69 = pleural effusion above the diaphragm

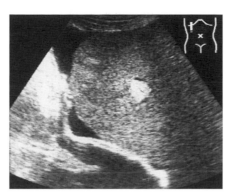

Fig. 109.1 a

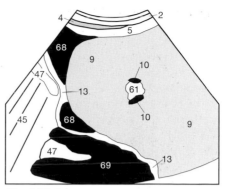

Fig. 109.1 b

Answer to Question on the Upper GI Series on Page 64

The contrast medium (white) is in the posteriorly located fundus and pylorus/duodenum – a result of gravitation. The anteriorly located body of the stomach is easily evaluated with the help of the double contrast visualization. This distribution of contrast medium indicates that the patient is supine. If the examiner wants to evaluate the gastric fundus, the patient must be brought in the upright position or turned on the right side – so that the contrast medium can leave the fundus.

To visualize the duodenal bulb, the patient must be turned on the left side. Please remember that the patient has to be NPO for an upper GI series and that gastric peristalsis might need to be pharmacologically paralyzed (side effects of intravenously injected methylscopolamine!) to achieve a reliable result. It is advisable to tell the patient beforehand to try not to burp and release the air produced by the effervescent powder – how else can he know if he is not told?

Answer to Question on Page 79

Figure 75.2b illustrates the anatomic orientation of endovaginal images. The right border of the image is posterior.

Therefore, the posteriorly gravitated blood clot is on the right border of the image in Fig. 79.3.

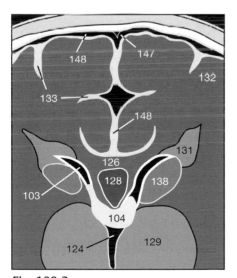

Fig. 109.2

Answer to Figure 103.1 (Question 2):

Sonographic section:
Intracerebral coronal section at the level of the foramen of Monro (144)
Structures:
Lateral ventricle (103), 3rd ventricle (124), thalamus (129), cerebral sulci (133), choroid plexus (104), grey matter (132), periventricular white matter (131), corpus callosum (126), head of the caudate nucleus (138)
CSF spaces:

Interhemispheric space (146)	< 6 mm
Sinocortical width (147)	< 3 mm
Craniocortical width (148)	< 4 mm
Width of the 3rd ventricle (124)	< 10 mm
Width of the lateral ventricle (frontal horn)	< 13 mm

Normal variant:
Cavum septi pellucidi (128)

On the pages with the quiz questions, I offered you an approach to memorize sectional anatomy by means of drawing exercises. How does it work?

It works with surprisingly little effort: It is based on the idea to draw and annotate specific standard planes from memory (in the cafeteria, e.g., on a napkin, during coffee break or at night on any piece of paper) with long intervals in between. Do not spend more than two minutes on such an exercise!

Thereafter, you fill in your gaps with the help of the diagram templates copied from this page. You just have to carry your copies with you (in your lab coat pocket?). Only after this exercise has faded from your short-term memory (> 2 to 4 hours), you should begin a new attempt. You will be surprised how few exercises it takes to master the sectional anatomy – as long as you approach these tasks with the spirit of self-improvement. Good luck with your efforts...

Sagittal section of the UA left paramedian (AO)

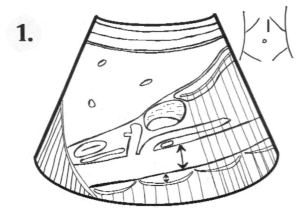

Sagittal section of the UA right paramedian (IVC)

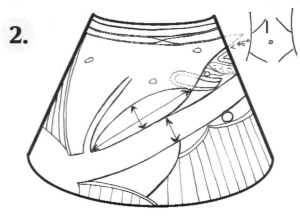

Para-iliac oblique section of the LA

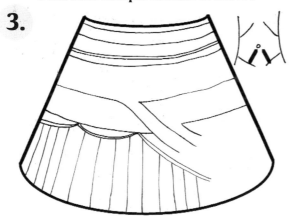

Transverse section of the UA (celiac axis)

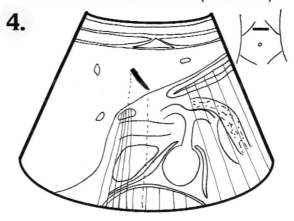

Transverse section of the UA (renal vein crossing)

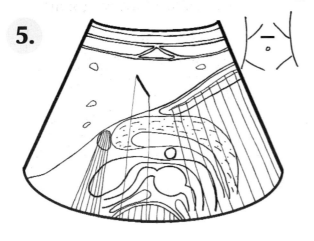

Right oblique section of the UA (porta hepatis)

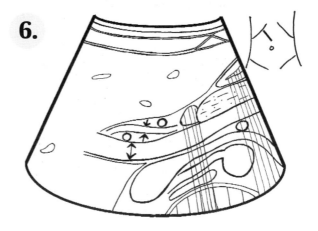

Of course, these diagrams represent idealized situations showing structures usually not found in the same plane in a real patient. This doesn't matter, tough. What matters is your sovereign ability to find, for instance, the pancreas or the origins of the renal artery in obese patients with limited sonographic visibility. Most patients are visual learners – and most likely you will be one as well.

With time, you will acquire a "visual template" of the expected findings (= normal findings) of every standard plane and you will immediately notice any deviation ("something doesn't look right here"). That is the goal. You should even go one step further by adding the normal values where you find arrows pointing in opposite directions (⟷) – this way you will memorize the normal values as well.

On this page we added a minor mistake for the advanced reader. Can you find it?

Right subcostal oblique section (hepatic veins)

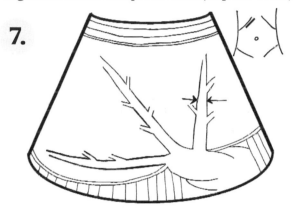

7.

Transhepatic longitudinal section right kidney

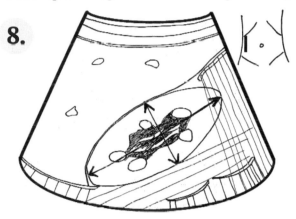

8.

Transverse section right kidney / IVC

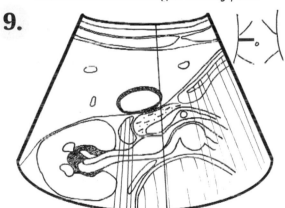

9.

High section of the left flank (spleen)

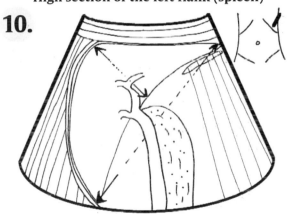

10.

Suprapubic sagittal section median (urinary bladder / uterus)

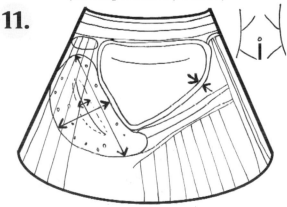

11.

Suprapubic transverse section (urinary bladder / prostate gland)

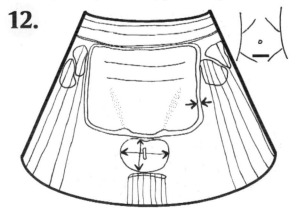

12.

When communicating with experienced colleagues, the "novice" is occasionally confounded when deciding which terminology to use to describe findings in an efficient and exact way. This brief review should be of help until you have become more familiar with the common terms.

A   General description of the sonographic morphology of an abnormality:

Section plane?	Name section plane (see front cover flap) Visualization of the lesion in longitudinal or transverse diameter?
How large?	Stated in mm or cm. Important for serial examination: Determination of progression or regression, e.g., during therapy
Where?	Location, laterality, position relative to other organs and vessels, e.g., central, hilar ⟷ peripheral, subcapsular, wall-based
Number?	Possible lesions: single, multiple or diffuse pattern
Echogenicity?	Anechoic (= homogeneous fluid), hypoechoic or hyperechoic (possibly relative to surroundings)
Shape?	E.g., round, oval, spherical ⟷ stellate, wedge-shaped, geographic, irregular, clubbed
Demarcation?	Sharp (more likely benign) ⟷ indistinct (= evidence of infiltration, e.g., in inflammation or malignancy)
Echo texture?	Homogeneous ⟷ heterogeneous; fine granular ⟷ coarse; septated; Recently also: elastic deformity (in special interrogation technique)
Acoustic phenomena?	Acoustic shadow, edge effect, total reflection, acoustic enhancement, section-thickness/mirror/side-lobe artifacts, reverberation artifacts
Expansion?	Displacement/infiltration of adjacent structures/vessels? Caution: space-occupying effects also possible with benign cysts, therefore not necessarily equated with malignancy

B   Useful terms, in alphabetical order   (⇨ application, possible meaning)

Ampullary	Developmental variant of the renal pelvis (⇨ can mimic obstruction)	Density	Sometimes incorrectly used term: the echo genicity of a tissue seen on the sonographic image has little in common with its physical density
Anechoic	Black (⇨ homogeneous fluids: blood, urine, bile, cyst contents, and pericardial / pleural effusion)		
Artifact	Products not indicative of actual structural relationships	Depth compensation	Depth-controlled gain adjustment
Bulging	Smooth convex expansion / displacement of adjacent structures (⇨ tumors)	Diffuse	Distribution pattern, e.g., of increased echogenicity
Capsule line	Thin, hyperechoic organ outline (⇨ absent in cirrhosis)	Dissection	Complication of (⇨ aortic aneurysm)
Cockade	Target phenomenon (⇨ intestinal invagination, DD: inflammatory mural thickening of the intestine)	Distinct	Demarcation (⇨ benign criterion)
		Double-barrel phenomenon	Immediate vicinity of two anechoic ductal structures in the hepatic parenchyma (⇨ dilation of intrahepatic biliary ducts parallel to the portal vein branches)
Comet tail	Artifact induced by resonance behind pulmonary/intestinal air	Eccentric	Asymmetrically wall-based (⇨ e.g., intravascular location of a thrombus)
Concentric	Pericentrally arranged in a vessel (⇨ thrombosis, calcification)	Echogenicity	Brightness of the pixels (increases with number of impedance jumps)
Curtain trick	Breathing instruction (⇨ to improve the visualization of the spleen)	Ectasia	Dilation of the lumen of the abdominal aorta > 2.5 - 3.0 cm

Edge effect	Phenomenon behind edge of the gallbladder and cysts
Fluke-like	Typical configuration of the celiac axis on transverse section
FNH	Focal nodular hyperplasia of the liver
Focal	A focally confined lesion
Focal zone	Volume lying within the highest vertical resolution
Forced inspiration	Respiratory maneuver ($\Rightarrow$ vena cava collapse test)
Gain	Amplification of received signal used for image display
Halo	Hypoechoic rim of a lesion ($\Rightarrow$ typical of, e.g., hepatic metastases)
Haustration	Localized bulging (typical outline of the colon)
Heterogenous	Irregular distribution or echo texture
Hilus fat sign	Sign of a benign nodal enlargement
Hyperechoic	Bright (e.g., fatty infiltration of parenchymal organs)
Hypoechoic	Dark, few echoes ($\Rightarrow$ muscles, subcutaneous fat, parenchyma)
Impedance jump	Echo-inducing interphase between tissue layers of different sound velocity
Indistinctness	Indistinct demarcation ($\Rightarrow$ criterion of infiltration in malignancy / inflammation)
Infiltration	Spreading into neighboring structures ($\Rightarrow$ sign of malignancy / inflammation)
Iris aperture phenomenon	Typical contrast enhancement of hepatic hemangiomas in dynamic spiral CT
Jet phenomenon	Ureteric urine propulsion into the urinary bladder; in color Doppler sonography: $\Rightarrow$ intra- and poststenotic flow acceleration
Kinking	Twisted or curled upon itself ($\Rightarrow$ aortic aneurysm)
L / T ratio	Longitudinal diameter divided by the transverse diameter ($\Rightarrow$ determining benign or malignant enlargement of LN)
Liquefaction	Generally anechoic ($\Rightarrow$ e.g., in the center of abscesses, metastases)
LN	Lymph node
Multifocal	Several foci in one organ
Necrosis	Hypoechoic, usually central liquefaction ($\Rightarrow$ abscess, metastasis)
Nodular	Distribution pattern in the form of nodules
Non-propulsive peristalsis	Alternating forward and backward peristalsis, e.g., of the intestinal contents
Nutcracker	Phenomenon of arterial compression of the left renal vein by aorta and superior mesenteric artery
Pennate pattern	Parallel stripes ($\Rightarrow$ characteristic of muscles, e.g., psoas muscle)
Perifocal	Rim around a lesion
Plaque	Hyperechoic calcified zone along vascular walls
Pneumobilia	Air in the biliary ducts ($\Rightarrow$ S / P papillotomy / abscess)

PP index	Parenchyma-pelvic index ($\Rightarrow$ evaluation of the kidneys)
Predilection	Preferred location of a lesion / abnormality
Pruned	Sudden change in caliber of the portal vein branches ($\Rightarrow$ cirrhosis)
Pseudocysts	($\Rightarrow$ Complication of pancreatitis)
Pulsation	Uniphasic ($\Rightarrow$ arteries, e.g., aorta) Biphasic ($\Rightarrow$ veins, e.g., inferior vena cava)
Rarefaction	Less areal density of vessels ($\Rightarrow$ e.g., cirrhosis)
Respecting	Deference to vessels speaks against infiltrative growth ($\Rightarrow$ benign criterion)
Reverberation	Repetitive echoes (artifact)
Rounding	Changed configuration of an organ ($\Rightarrow$ rounded edge of the liver in cirrhosis)
Scalloped	Series of circle segments, cauliflower-like ($\Rightarrow$ e.g., exophytic tumor configuration in the stomach and urinary bladder)
Section thickness artifact	Indistinct delineation of a hollow viscus wall obliquely hit by the sound beam
Septate	Anechoic hollow spaces traversed by echogenic lines ($\Rightarrow$ cysts, e.g., cystic ovarian tumors; aortic dissection)
Side-lobe artifact	$\Rightarrow$ Occurs in anechoic structures next to strong reflectors
Sludge	Sedimented echogenic matter in the gallbladder
Sound beam lobe	Finite thickness of the sound beam $\Rightarrow$ section thickness artifact
Spoke wheel-like	Echogenicity pattern ($\Rightarrow$ FNH of the liver) ($\Rightarrow$ septation in ecchinococcal cysts)
Starry skies	Multiple hyperechoic splenic lesions ($\Rightarrow$ e.g., tuberculous involvement of the spleen)
Stenosis	Narrowing of a vessel or intestine
Stent	Tube implanted to relieve a stenosis
String of pearls	$\Rightarrow$ Arrangement of the medullary pyramids along the cortical-caliceal junction $\Rightarrow$ dilation of the pancreatic duct in pancreatitis
Target sign	Concentric arrangement of alternating echogenicity ($\Rightarrow$ e.g., small bowel intussusception)
Thinned parenchymal cortex	($\Rightarrow$ typical for damaged renal parenchyma)
Total reflection	Black shadow behind bones and air
Trackball	A device that controls the cursor on the display
Triangular	Typical three-cornered configuration of organ infarcts
Vena cava collapse test	Maneuver using forced inspiration ($\Rightarrow$ in suspected right heart decompensation)
Wall thickness	Sonographic finding ($\Rightarrow$ of hollow viscus or vessels)
Wedge-shaped	Increased echogenicity of the parenchyma ($\Rightarrow$ typical configuration of an infarct)

The following list contains terms that are applicable to certain organ systems. First, a description of the location is provided, followed by typical sonographic changes with possible inference as to the underlying abnormality.

Finally, any specific issue related to the organ is listed. This section is suitable as a short and timesaving review.

Liver
Spatial Terms
- Subdiaphragmatic, subcapsular ↔ perihilar, central; name segmental location (not only lobar), periportal, parahepatic, focal ↔ diffuse

Typical Morphology
⇨ Possible Diagnosis
- Diffuse increase in echogenicity
  ⇨ Fatty liver
- Diffuse loss of sound penetration with depth
  ⇨ Fatty liver
- Geographic, sharply marginated differences in echogenicity around the gallbladder fossa or near the portal vein
  ⇨ Focally increased or decreased fatty infiltration
- Spherical anechoic and sharply marginated lesions with edge effect and posterior acoustic enhancement
  ⇨ Benign cysts
- Cameral cyst with septation
  ⇨ Echinococcal cyst
  (splenic involvement)
- Singular or multiple lesions with hypoechoic rim (= halo)
  ⇨ Metastases
- Spherical hyperechoic and sharply marginated lesion without a halo
  ⇨ Hemangioma
- Double barrel phenomenon along portal veins
  ⇨ Dilated intrahepatic bile ducts
- Intraductal hyperechoic and oval lesions with acoustic shadowing
  ⇨ Gallstones or pneumobilia
- Absent capsule line, peripherally rarefied vessels, rounded organ edges and pruned portal vein branches
  ⇨ Cirrhosis (only late in the disease also a shrunken liver)

Specific Issues
- Clarification of DD with contrast harmonic imaging and elastographic methods

- Spiral CT: Dynamic study with typical contrast enhancement pattern diagnostic of hemangioma: "iris phenomenon"

Gallbladder
Spatial Terms
- Endoluminal, wall-based, infundibular, fundal

Typical Morphology
⇨ Possible Diagnosis
- Hypoechoic, multilayered and edematous wall thickening, possibly with perifocal "ascites"
  ⇨ Acute cholecystitis
- Intraluminal, hyperechoic sedimentation phenomenon
  ⇨ Sludge (DD: section thickness, reverberation and side lobe artifacts)
- Hyperechoic, spherical to oval lesion with posterior acoustic shadowing
  ⇨ Cholecystolithiasis
- Focal wall thickening or wall-adherent hyperechoic lesion without acoustic shadowing
  ⇨ Polyp

Spleen
Spatial Terms
- Subdiaphragmatic, subcapsular ↔ central, perihilar; perisplenic, parasplenic

Typical Morphology
⇨ Possible Diagnosis
- Rounded organ shape
  ⇨ Splenomegaly with viral infection, lymphoma or portal hypertension
- Triangular / wedge-shaped area of decreased echogenicity
  ⇨ Suspicious for infarct => color Doppler sonography
- Heterogeneous – patchy parenchyma
  ⇨ Suspicious for lymphomatous infiltration
- Parasplenic round space-occupying lesion with echogenicity identical to spleen
  ⇨ Accessory spleen, LN
- Hypoechoic, bandlike discontinuity of the parenchyma, possibly with subcapsular hypoechoic fluid
  ⇨ Suspicious for splenic rupture (free abdominal fluid?)

Pancreas
Spatial Terms
- Head, uncinate process, body, tail, disseminated, peripancreatic, lesser bursa

Typical Morphology
⇨ Possible Diagnosis
- Diffuse increase in echogenicity
  ⇨ Lipomatosis
- Hypoechoic edematous enlargement with pain on graded pressure of the transducer, possible detection of peripancreatic anechoic fluid
  ⇨ Acute pancreatitis
- Organ atrophy with focal hyperechoic calcifications with acoustic shadowing, possible irregular dilation of the pancreatic duct
  ⇨ Chronic pancreatitis
- Anechoic, cystic hollow spaces in the pancreatic region
  ⇨ Pseudocyst
  (DD fluid-filled bowel loop)

Specific Issues
- Possibility of endosonographic visualization from the stomach

Adrenal Glands
Typical Morphology
⇨ Possible Diagnosis
- Uni- or bilateral, hypoechoic enlargement
  ⇨ Adenoma DD metastasis

Specific Issues
- Clarification of DD by means of dynamic spiral CT (contrast enhancement wash-out curve)

Kidneys
Spatial Terms
- (Para)pelvic, perihilar ↔ subcapsular, parenchymal, cortical, pericapsular, polar, perirenal, at the PP junction, uni- / bilateral; do not forget laterality (body marker)

Typical Morphology
⇨ Possible Diagnosis
- Homogeneous, anechoic, round to oval and sharply demarcated lesion with posterior sound enhancement
  ⇨ Cyst
- Homogenous, hyperechoic, sharply demarcated and spherical lesion
  ⇨ Angiolipoma
- String-of-pearl-like arranged at the PP junction, hypoechoic, spherical lesions without posterior acoustic enhancement
  ⇨ Physiologic medullary pyramids
- Hypoechoic clubbing / prominent pelvis
  ⇨ Urinary obstruction (DD pelvic cyst, ampullary renal pelvis)
- Thinned cortex with PPI < normal and renal size < 10 cm
  ⇨ Renal atrophy

- Heterogeneous space-occupying lesion with expansion
  ⇨ Suspicious for malignancy
- Hyperechoic, wedge-shaped area in the cortex
  ⇨ Suspicious for infarct

Specific Issues
- Clarification of the DD with density measurement on spiral CT and perfusion pattern of color-coded Doppler ultrasound
- Ectopic kidney, horseshoe kidney
- Accessory renal arteries

Upper GI Tract
Spatial Terms
- Intraluminal, wall-based, for bowel also state the abdominal quadrant

Typical Morphology
⇨ Possible Diagnosis
- Target sign (concentric formation of alternating echogenicity)
  ⇨ Intestinal invagination
- Focal, hypoechoic wall thickening with discontinuity of the mural layers
  ⇨ suspicious for malignancy
  DD lymphoma: rather disseminated than focal

Specific Issues
- Optional hypotonic visualization of the gastric wall with water as anechoic intraluminal medium
- Possible endosonography (gastric and rectal wall)
- Triggering of peristalsis with rapidly alternating pressure on the transducer

Urinary Bladder
Spatial Terms
- Intraluminal, wall-based, intra-, extra- and paravesical, bladder floor, bladder roof

Typical Morphology
⇨ Possible Diagnosis
- Hyperechoic gravitational matter
  ⇨ Grist, hematoma
- Diffuse, hypoechoic wall thickening
  ⇨ Cystitis
- Focal wall thickening, possibly growing as polypoid projection into the lumen
  ⇨ Suspicious for malignancy
- Paravesical, spherical, anechoic and sharply marginated formation
  ⇨ Bladder diverticulum
- Spherical, hyperechoic intraluminal line
  ⇨ Balloon of Foley catheter
  (rare DD: ureterocele in children)

- Suddenly appearing linear intraluminal heterogeneity
  ⇨ Jet phenomenon representing urine propelled from the ureteral ostium by ureteral peristalsis

Specific Issues
- Clamping of any indwelling catheter to fill the lumen for adequate evaluation of the bladder wall

Vessels and Retroperitoneum
Spatial Terms
- Para-, retro-, pre-aortal or -caval, interaortocaval, prevertebral, retrocrural, mesenterial, para-iliac, inguinal, cervical

Typical Morphology
⇨ Possible Diagnosis
- Endoluminal matter of various echogenicity
  ⇨ Thrombus
- Diameter of thrombosed vein more than twice of that of the accompanying artery
  ⇨ Indicative of acute thrombosis (<10 days)
- Dilated aortic lumen containing a hyperechoic membrane
  ⇨ dissected aortic aneurysm
- Hypoechoic ovoid structure next to a vessel
  ⇨ Typical of lymph node (LN)
- Ovoid LN (L / T ratio > 2) with hilar fat sign
  ⇨ benign criteria of LN
- Spherical LN (L / T ratio ~ 1) with homogeneous hypoechogenicity without hilus fat sign
  ⇨ Typical of lymphoma (perfusion pattern to be determined by color-coded Doppler sonography)

Specific Issues
- Often additional information with color-coded Doppler sonography

Thyroid Gland
Spatial Terms
- Isthmus, lobes (state laterality), subcapsular, upper or lower pole

Typical Morphology
⇨ Possible Diagnosis
- Isoechoic nodular lesions with hypoechoic rim
  ⇨ Typical of adenoma
- Cystic anechoic lesion, often multifocal
  ⇨ Nodular transformation induced by iodine deficiency
- Hypoechoic nodular lesions
  ⇨ Suspicious for malignancy if scintigraphically nonfunctioning ("cold")

- Diffuse hypoechogenicity of the normally more hyperechoic parenchyma
  ⇨ Hashimoto thyroiditis
- Thyroid enlargement with indistinctly demarcated hypoechoic areas within otherwise normal echogenicity
  ⇨ Subacute thyroiditis de Quervain

Specific Issues
- Interpretation often together with scintigraphy and color-coded Doppler sonography

C Checklists

The third part of this review comprises the checklists, which are not repeated here to save space. They are listed on the pocket-size cards or on the following pages:

Index	Template of Normal Ultrasound Report

Template of Normal Ultrasound Report

The subsequent text should serve as guideline for a normal ultrasound report:

Template of a normal report for patient _____
Date of birth _____

The examination was performed without / with contrast enhancer with a _____ MHz transducer / with following additional techniques: THI / CHI / SonoCT® _____

Retroperitoneum:
The retroperitoneum is well seen without evidence of any lymphadenopathy or other pathologic space-occupying lesions. Aorta and inferior vena cava are unremarkable.

Pancreas:
The parenchyma is homogeneous without evidence of focal lesions or inflammation. The size of the pancreas is within the range of normal / enlarged, with the head measuring ___ cm, the body ___ cm and the tail ___ cm. The pancreatic duct is normal measuring ____ mm in diameter / is not visualized / _____. (*Delete non-applicable statements.*)

Liver:
The liver is normal in size and configuration and exhibits a smooth surface. The parenchyma has a normal homogeneous echogenicity without evidence of focal space-occupying lesions. Intrahepatic biliary ducts and vessels appear normal.

Gallbladder / Biliary Ducts:
The gallbladder is average in size and configuration and without evidence of inflammatory wall thickening, stones or sludge. The biliary ducts are not dilated. The distal common bile duct is well / partially visualized to _____.

Adrenal Glands:
Both adrenal glands are unremarkable without evidence of a mass.

Kidneys:
Both kidneys are well visualized, show normal respiratory mobility and are normal in size, with the right kidney measuring ____ cm and the left kidney ____ cm in length. The parenchyma is homogeneous and of normal width bilaterally, with a PP index of ____ on the right and _____ on the left. No evidence of calcifications, hydronephrosis or space-occupying lesions.

Spleen:
The spleen is normal in size for the patient's age, measuring _____ cm in length and _____ cm in width, and exhibits a homogeneous parenchyma. No sonographic evidence of focal lesions. The application of _____ brings out _____.

Peritoneal Cavity:
No evidence of free fluid.

Gastrointestinal Tract:
The gastric wall thickness is within the normal range, measuring _____ mm. No evidence of focal wall thickness of the stomach, small intestines or colon. Normal peristaltic was observed.

Urinary Bladder:
The wall is smoothly outlined and normal in width, measuring _____ mm. Normal postvoid residual volume of ____ ml. No evidence of stones, diverticula or ureterocele.

Reproductive Organs:
Reproductive Organs:
The **uterus** is normal for the patient's age, measuring ____ x ____ cm. The width of endometrium is _____ mm when measuring both layers together. No evidence of retained secretion or focal lesions. No evidence of free fluid in the cul-de-sac. The ovaries are well visualized / not visualized on the (right / left) and are normal in size, with the right ovary measuring ____ x ____ cm and the left ovary ____ x ____ cm.
The **prostate gland** is homogeneous and normal in size, measuring ____ x ____ x ____ cm. No evidence of focal lesions or calcifications. The seminal vesicles are unremarkable.

Conclusion:
Unremarkable examination of the abdomen and retroperitoneum. (Don't forget to address the clinical question; *delete non-applicable statement*)
Remarks:_____

This updated and expanded second English edition could not have been realized without the support of numerous helpers. Since 1991, more than 3,000 course participants, scores of readers and 100 course instructors have contributed to the continuing optimization of this workbook in systematic evaluations with feedback and constructive criticism. I wish to thank them all.

My special gratitude goes to Mrs. Susanne Kniest for the excellent graphic rendering of many new sketches and to Mrs. Inger Juergens for the book's layout. Siemens Medical Solutions, Mr. Gert Hetzel and W. Krzos (Fig. 10.3) and my colleagues C.F. Dietrich (Fig. 38.4) and D. Becker (Fig. 10.2, 10.3) provided several images illustrating the value of new techniques. My colleague Tatjana Reihs provided most of the obstetrical and gynecological images.

I cordially thank my wife Stefanie for her critical review and additional creative suggestions. Finally, I wish to mention my teaching sonographers in this teaching project and to honor their willingness to participate in intensive continuing education by making a worthfull contribution to the success of the entire project.

Currently, they include Nadine Abanador, Arne Gerber, Rolf Hanrath M.D., Markus Hollenbeck M.D., Jae-Hyuk Hwang M.D., Lars Kamper M.D., Stefanie Keymel, Janine Metten M.D., Sebastian Pohle, Alexander Rosen, Ralf Rulands, Stefan Schmidt and Maren Totzauer.

Matthias Hofer, M.D., MPH
Diagnostic Radiologist
Director Medical Education Pilot Project
Institutes of Diagnostic Radiology and Anatomy II
Heinrich-Heine University Duesseldorf, Germany